COMMUNITY ORGANIZATION AND SOCIAL ADMINISTRATION: ADVANCES, TRENDS, AND EMERGING PRINCIPLES

Terry Mizrahi, PhD
John Morrison, DSW
Editors

SOME ADVANCE REVIEWS

"The systematic investigations reported throughout this volume and the specific practice prescriptions drawn from these inquiries are a refreshing addition to a literature that has tended to be long on abstract concepts and short on guidance for practitioners. This book will be welcomed by those who teach and do scholarship on community organization, planning, and social change. There are not only several original and instructive research studies, but some impressive case studies that will provide good grist for the teaching-learning mill."

Rino J. Patti, DSW
Dean, USC Scho~~ol of Social Work~~

"This book could not be ~~more timely, nor~~ more important. It brings together chapters on ~~original research~~ and theorizing on strategies of coalition-building ~~and management,~~ strategies of advocacy and grassroots orga~~nizing, evaluation~~ of social change efforts, and the role of po~~litical action~~ ~~in~~ ~~social~~ work curriculum. The enormous value of this ~~book is that~~ it tells us — in sophisticated, vivid, and pragmatic wa~~ys — how~~ to fight back."

Richard A. Cloward, PhD
Professor, Columbia University School of Social Work

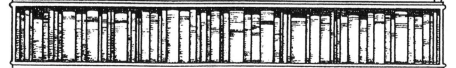

"This edited work is an artful blend of classic theory along with contemporary and critical topics for macro practice in the 1990s. The organization of the text indicates quickly the span of its content from community practice, planning, and administration to political activism. Of equal importance is the inclusion of topics usually absent from macro-practice texts, including coalition building, agency administration in retrenchment, and feminist analysis. This collection would be an extremely valuable addition to any macro-practice course."

Karen S. Haynes, PhD, MSW
Dean and Professor
Graduate School of Social Work
University of Houston

"Social workers in a variety of agencies as well as public health and other human services workers will find this book of readings about the advances that have developed in the past decade stimulating and informative. Although there is a tendency by many to view macro-practice in social work from a unidimensional perspective, these papers demonstrate the utility of a multi-disciplinary approach, as well as the importance of a perspective that advocates approaches based on both theory and acknowledgement of how social values influence practice."

Rosemary Sarri, PhD
Professor of Social Work
University of Michigan

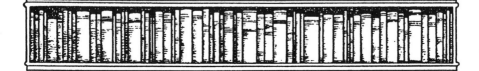

Community Organization and Social Administration

Advances, Trends, and Emerging Principles

Community
Organization
and
Social Administration
Advances, Trends and Emerging Principles

Terry Mizrahi, PhD
John Morrison, DSW
Editors

The Haworth Press
New York • London • Norwood (Australia)

Community Organization and Social Administration: Advances, Trends, and Emerging Principles is supplement #4 to *Administration in Social Work* (ISSN 0364-3107). It is not supplied as part of the subscription to the journal, but is available from the publisher at an additional charge.

The Haworth Press, Inc., 10 Alice Street, Binghamton, NY 13904-1580

Library of Congress Cataloging-in-Publication Data

Community organization and social administration : advances, trends, and emerging principles / Terry Mizrahi, John Morrison, editors.
  p. cm.
  Includes bibliographical references.
  ISBN 1-56024-277-9 (acid free paper).
  1. Community development—United States. 2. Social work administration—United States. 3. Community organization—United States. I. Mizrahi, Terry. II. Morrison, John D.
HN90.C6C6625   1992
307.1′4′0973—dc20   92-8960
                                                                        CIP

CONTENTS

PART 4: ENHANCING EDUCATION IN COMMUNITY ORGANIZATION AND SOCIAL ADMINISTRATION

ABOUT THE EDITORS

Terry Mizrahi, PhD, is Professor at the Hunter College School of Social Work and Director of the Education Center for Community Organizing (ECCO). An experienced community organizer and advocate, she has research, writing, and consultation expertise in interdisciplinary collaboration and coalition building, health organizing, health policy, and patients' rights. She is the author of several books, including *Getting Rid of Patients: Contradictions in the Socialization of Physicians* (Rutgers University Press, 1986) and is co-editor of *Computers for Social Change and Community Organizing* (The Haworth Press, 1991). She is the secretary of the National Association of Social Workers, and was vice-president of the New York City Chapter. She is also membership secretary of the Association on Community Organization and Social Administration.

John Morrison, DSW, is Professor at Aurora University School of Social Work in Illinois where he teaches courses in policy, community organization, and administration. Dr. Morrison's academic interests and publications are in the areas of neighborhood development, intergroup relations, and issues related to older adults. He has conducted a number of studies in community development and planning, and served as Assistant Commissioner of the New York City Community Development Agency, and as Director of community centers in Brooklyn. Dr. Morrison has been a board member, officer, and consultant to a wide range of organizations.

Acknowledgments

The editors would like to thank Simon Slavin, Editor of *Administration in Social Work* for his generous support of ACOSA over the years. We are particularly appreciative for his leadership in this new venture.

Special thanks are due the people who developed the ACOSA publication proposal or served as reviewers for this book: Eleanor Brilliant, William Buffum, Stephen Burghardt, Michael Fabricant, Audrey Faulkner, Joan Hashimi, Bruce Jansson, Paul Keys, Jean Kruzich, Paul Kurzman, Armand Lauffer, Ray MacNair, Jacqueline Mondros, Michael Reisch, Felix Rivera, Maria Roberts-De-Gennaro, Herbert Rubin, Andrea Savage, Marie Weil, Stanley Wenocur, Stephen Wernet, Scott Wilson. Thanks are due, too, to Albert E. Wilkerson, Assistant Editor of *Administration in Social Work*, for his technical editing work on the final manuscript.

Introduction

Terry Mizrahi, PhD
John Morrison, DSW

It is with great pleasure and excitement that we introduce *Community Organization and Social Administration: Advances, Trends, and Emerging Principles*, a publication of the Association on Community Organization and Social Administration (ACOSA). ACOSA was developed from a series of annual symposia on community organization and social administration affiliated with the annual program meetings of the Council on Social Work Education (Weil & Kruzich, 1990). Over the years, selected papers were published in special issues of different journals (Leibowitz, 1982; Burghardt & Seckel, 1982; Gruber, 1983; Austin, 1984; Reisch & Wenocur, 1986; Neugeboren, 1987; Weil & Kruzich, 1990). In the late 1980s interest grew in producing an independent journal devoted to community and agency-based practice. After exploring several options, ACOSA, which had been formally established by then, was offered the best of both worlds: a chance to affiliate with a well-known and respected journal, *Administration in Social Work*, while editing its own independently produced book annually. The articles in this premier volume were selected from peer reviewed papers, either presented at annual ACOSA symposia or from a separate call.

ACOSA is a growing organization whose mission is to strengthen and develop macro-practice within social work, link educators with practitioners, and contribute to the advancement and synthesis of

---

Dr. Mizrahi is Professor and Director of the Education Center for Community Organizing at Hunter College School of Social Work, The City University of New York, 129 East 79th Street, New York, NY 10021. Dr. Morrison is Professor, School of Social Work, Aurora University, 347 S. Gladstone Street, Aurora, IL 60506.

1

theory and practice. It is our hope that this volume will help achieve these goals.

THE GLOBAL CONTEXT

The development of this volume, *Community Organization and Social Administration: Advances, Trends, and Emerging Principles,* coincides with our entering the final decade of the twentieth century. The year 1990 truly seemed like the best of times and the worst of times. Unprecedented changes in the world politic occurred which signaled the end of the "cold war." Historic changes in South Africa were taking place to end apartheid. For the first time in almost half a century, the potential for living in peace without the threat of major war seemed possible. Organizers called for a "peace dividend" to convert resources from military to human services.

Declining social conditions made such a dividend seem long overdue. Infant mortality rates began to rise in some communities, the gap widened between rich and poor and between peoples of color and white Americans. Homeless people appeared in ever-increasing numbers, and the infra-structure of large urban areas continued to decay. The Bush administration continued the economic and political conservatism of the Reagan years, eroding if not cutting, housing, health and human services, and family policy. There were great holes in the safety net (Burghardt & Fabricant, 1987). A pessimism began to pervade the land as an official government announcement of a recession rang in the New Year 1991.

As this book goes to press in Fall 1992, the United States continues to be in a long-lasting recession accompanied by rising levels of unemployment. Policies that limit public assistance, Medicaid, and other health and human services to the poor and working class are being passed in Congress and in many state legislatures. The public confidence in our nation's, and especially President Bush's ability to solve long-term economic and social problems is at an all-time low. The prospect of a "peace dividend" resulting from the end of the "Cold War" seems distant now.

Social Work Activism

Yet even in these hard times, visions and strategies for improving social conditions and for strengthening families and communities are found in this book. Each of the eleven papers describes ways that social workers and other progressive community and human services leaders are engaged in social change efforts. The practice principles offered to organizers, administrators, planners, and educators are grounded in the real world of political and social activism. At the same time, many of the writers have sought to identify and integrate theory into their data-based findings. The conceptual base of practice is also evident in attempts to develop and apply theory to administrative practice.

THE CONTRIBUTORS AND THEIR CONTRIBUTIONS

We are pleased that a majority of the authors are women, the highest percentage found in any ACOSA-initiated special issue. Of the twenty-two authors contributing to this volume, seven are either practitioners or administrators of community programs connected with academic institutions. We would like to encourage and attract more field-based articles and greater collaboration between the university and the community, modeled on some of the works produced here (e.g., Starr & Schachter; Mizrahi & Rosenthal; Mary et al.; and Chavis et al.).

Most of the papers document how practitioners and educators are addressing a variety of specialized fields such as school social work (Starr & Schachter), mental health (Friesen; Wernet), planning (MacNair), organizing (Mizrahi & Rosenthal; Mondros & Wilson) and management (McMurtry et al.).

The Response to the New Political Realities: Moving from the 1980s to the 1990s

A number of the earlier ACOSA-initiated volumes spoke to the funding crisis brought about by Reaganomics and a resurgence of conservative policy. While there is a continuing concern about the future found in the current group of papers, there is also a greater sense that concerted action and thoughtful leadership can be effective in maintaining and developing services and progressive policies. The regressive climate of the 1980s was an impetus for some creative and proactive organizing, planning, managing, and developing programs as reported by MacNair; Starr and Schachter; Pine et al.; and Mizrahi and Rosenthal. In other instances the works focus upon capturing and utilizing the few still existing progressive programs, policies and movements such as in mental health (Friesen; Wernet), feminism (Halseth), and community development (Chavis et al.).

All of the authors identify, and some address directly, the larger political and economic context in which their work is embedded. While most of the articles identify real obstacles to building and sustaining organizations resulting from the harsh survival realities of the 80s, many of the authors also describe and analyze the ways some groups have harnessed and creatively used limited resources (MacNair; McMurtry et al.; and Pine et al.). Most of the papers distinguish the larger external context from the environment that professionals can still influence, if not control. This enables practitioners to focus on effective strategies, skills, and leadership styles that can still make a difference (Mondros & Wilson; Mizrahi & Rosenthal; McMurtry et al.; Starr & Schachter; and Chavis et al.).

Organizational Survival and Development

Several of the papers deal with organizational survival: how to retain, sustain, and develop a program, organization, agency, or coalition in a time of cost containment and cutbacks. Utilizing practice-based research, Mondros and Wilson, and Mizrahi and Rosenthal, introduce a variety of strategies for organizers to use in maintaining the involvement and investment of people. Both Chavis et al. and Friesen describe the important role of technical assistance and enabling organizations in supporting consumer and grassroots groups. McMurtry et al. report the types of leadership and skill administrators use to avoid a reduction in client services to low or non-paying clients. Pine et al. present a modest, but effective attempt to maintain and develop the administration track at their school.

Empowerment

Empowerment was a theme of both the 1988 (Reisch & Wenocur) and 1990 (Weil & Kruzich) ACOSA-initiated publications. The editors of both these volumes also called for more specificity in use of the term empowerment. "Empowerment" can become an empty slogan through failure to identify how the process of empowerment specifically is achieved. The papers in this volume develop empowerment as an implicit theme. Many of the authors discuss principles and processes that do, in fact, empower clients, communities, and the professionals working on their behalf. Over the years, many of the symposia-based volumes have specifically called for development of both curricula and services that empower women and ethnic group members at the grassroots level. In this volume, Halseth suggests ways that a feminist perspective can enhance a macro-curriculum.

Coalitions

The importance of coalitions was recognized in past volumes as well as the current volume. In their introductory essay for the 1982 symposium papers, Burghardt and Seckel (1982) reported that "the necessity of more coalition building" was a strategic theme found in many of that issue's papers. Coalitions are one important way that practitioners and concerned citizens can achieve greater power and influence. The current volume features a number of papers that relate to coalition-building. The paper by Mizrahi and Rosenthal provides a number of principles for developing successful coalitions, and papers by Starr and Schachter, and Wernet and Friesen, demonstrate the impact that coalitions and inter-group collaborations can have on services.

Practice Advances: The Interdisciplinary Nature of Macro Social Work

Another continuing theme in past ACOSA issues, is the inherent connection between various macro-disciplines including community organization, planning, policy, and administration as well as the connection between the macro-disciplines and other components of social work. Austin (1984) traces the elaboration of the social work curriculum from three methods (casework, group work and community organization) into patterns that include micro-services to individuals and families and macro-services that focus on social development, planning, and policy analysis.

Burghardt and Seckel (1982) discuss the importance of better integration of macro-methods and theories and social work as a whole: "It may be that budget cuts and gutted programs are ironically forcing us into creatively joining once disparate factions into tighter fitting, more organically connected configurations that reflect the bare-boned realities of present day social welfare. Such creative applications, if they continue to develop at each symposium, may be part of social work's phoenix."

This volume seems to represent yet another step in bringing together the various macro-disciplines. In past years, papers from a particular symposium might appear in different journals depending on their practice focus. A single book, such as this one, that brings together community organization and administration papers now seems timely and appropriate. We have noted also the increasing interest in defining policy as a practice discipline and a move to introduce political content into all social work (Mary et al.). Reflecting the overall trend to reduce the distance between macro-disciplines, many of the papers here seem to span the macro-disciplines.

Theory and Values

The utilization and development of theory relevant to planning and social change is prevalent throughout this volume. These include organizational (McMurtry et al.; Mondros & Wilson), exchange and negotiation (Mizrahi & Rosenthal; Wernet), feminist (Halseth) and ecological and system theories (MacNair; Chavis et al.). Starr and Schachter, and Friesen, adapt and apply organizing concepts and principles to their current settings.

The importance of values as a guide to practice should be obvious. The value frame of most of the papers here is manifest: there is a clear concern for those with relatively little power and those people and communities with greatest needs.

Research Methodology

The papers also reflect a wide range of qualitative and quantitative methods to pursue systematic inquiry. Analyses of the strengths and limitations of data collection utilized by the authors further contribute to the research literature in macro-practice. Qualitative methods include the case study (Starr & Schachter; Friesen; Pine et al.; Wernet), in-depth interview (Mondros & Wilson); and focus groups (Mizrahi & Rosenthal). Quantitative methods include survey designs with known (McMurtry et al.; Mary et al.) and unknown (MacNair) subjects.

FOCUS ON THE FUTURE

Several important themes have been articulated by the authors that focus on the future. These are important for developing relevant educational programs that will produce committed and competent leaders in human services and community development in the 1990s. These are also critical for strengthening the effectiveness and increasing the satisfaction and productivity of practicing administrators and organizers. While these themes can be separately identified and learned, they are intertwined in practice.

Inter-organizational Coalition Building

The increasing importance of knowledge and skills in networking and coalition building. Whether in the public or private sector, at the neighborhood or national level, developing inter-organizational relationships and structures is essential for expanding or restructuring programs or policies.

Political Process

The understanding and application of the political system in its broadest sense, including the judicial, legislative, and regulatory structures and processes. Analyzing and utilizing pressure and electoral politics for achieving social service or social change goals will become increasingly critical.

Client and Community Participation

The renewed commitment to and skill in involving and retaining consumers and citizens in political advocacy and service planning. The momentum that began in the 1960s for citizen and client participation in shaping progressive social policies and programs is resurfacing in the 1990s with revived as well as new advocacy and planning models.

Resource Development

The continuing importance of skills in resource development including resource mobilization and management. Obtaining and retaining material and human resources through public and private fund raising methods are only part of the competencies needed to initiate, maintain and expand community-based organizations.

CONCLUSION

The above themes are not new. Many were articulated in earlier ACOSA-produced volumes: the role of politics in organizing, problems of localism and competing sectoral and regional interests (Burghardt & Seckel, 1982), and dark clouds of the social budget under the knife of Reaganomics (Gruber, 1983).

However, the dismantling of the ideology and reality of the nationally funded welfare state, with the resulting severe repercussions for state and local governments, was not predicted with the swiftness and intensity that it occurred. The skills and strategies needed to maintain a relevant systems-change perspective for all students, and macro-students in particular, was eloquently detailed by Karger and Reitmer (1983) almost ten years ago and is still relevant as we approach the 21st century.

While there is need for more research that synthesizes theory and practice, in the last decade we have developed greater confidence about our ability to deal with the future. We have moved from how we should respond to social conservatism, and even whether we could, to a more confident sense that we have a means to respond and can be ever more effective in the future.

Finally, this book demonstrates that the knowledge, commitment, and leadership to strengthen a social change perspective at the university and agency levels continue to thrive.

REFERENCES

Austin, D.M. Introduction to the special issue: Selected Papers on social administration. *Administration in Social Work*, 1984, *8*(3), 1-4.

Burghardt, S. & Seckel, J. Strategies for the 80s: Continuities and contradictions; responding to the attack on social welfare: New strategies for community organization and planning. *Social Development Issues*, 1982, *6*(3), 1-5.

Burghardt, S. & Fabricant, M. *Working Under the Safety Net*. Beverly Hills, CA: Sage, 1987.

Gruber, M.L. Introduction to the special issue. *Administration in Social Work*, 1983, *7*(3/4), 1-7.

Karger, J.H. & Reitmer, M.A. Community organization for the 1980s: Toward developing a new skills base within a political framework. *Social Development Issues*, 1983, *7*(2), 50-62.

Lebowitz, M.M. Introduction to the special issue: Practice issues in social administration, policy, and planning. *Administration in Social Work*, 1982, *6*(2/3), 1-6.

Neugeboren, B. Introduction to the special issue: legitimacy, effectiveness, and survival of macro education and practice. *Administration in Social Work*, 1987, *11*(2), 1-4.

Reisch, M. & Wenocur, S. Introduction: Symposium on community organization. *Journal of Sociology and Social Welfare*, 1986, *13*(3), 445-450.

Weil, M. & Kruzich, J. Introduction to the special issue: Empowerment issues in administrative and community practice. *Administration in Social Work*, 1990, *11*(20), 1-4.

PART 1: BUILDING AND SUSTAINING COMMUNITY INITIATIVES

Managing Dynamic Tensions in Social Change Coalitions

Terry Mizrahi, PhD
Beth B. Rosenthal, MS

INTRODUCTION

Professionals in social work, urban planning, and public administration are increasingly being called upon to participate in or give leadership to coalitions. Operating in increasingly complex environments, neighborhood-based and issue-targeting groups, social service directors, government officials, and business and labor leaders frequently need expert assistance in coalition-building. Human service leaders have a vital role to play in the promotion and

Dr. Mizrahi is Professor and Director of the Education Center for Community Organizing at Hunter College School of Social Work, The City University of New York, 129 East 79th Street, New York, NY 10021. Ms. Rosenthal is a Consultant and Trainer.

An earlier version of this paper was presented at the Association on Community Organization and Social Administration Symposium, Annual Program Meeting, Council on Social Work Education, Atlanta, Georgia, 1988.

use of coalitions, since they find themselves at the intersection between social problems and the services designed to address them. A better understanding of some of the dynamic tensions of coalitions may improve professional involvement in coalition functioning.

The coalition is a vital and increasingly utilized mechanism for collective organizing and policy formation. Coalitions are often a preferred vehicle for intergroup action because they promise to preserve the autonomy of member organizations while providing the necessary structure for unified effort. Enabling people to link special interests and share information and diverse expertise, coalitions are also means by which organizations can clarify their differences and incorporate various skills, levels of experience, and roles for participation.

Through coalitions, separate groups can develop a common language and ideology with which to shape a collective vision for progressive social change. Although the impetus for social change is often compelling, coalition-building is complex. Traditional community organizing and administrative skills are not automatically transferable to the development of coalitions, which require a greater degree of internal collaboration and planning.

This article focuses on the dynamic tensions inherent in coalitions, and describes how they are manifested and managed. It is part of our larger work in progress to synthesize what is known from both the theory and practice of coalition-building. This work includes other aspects of coalition-building such as stages of development, leadership techniques, decision-making methods, and elements of success and failure.

EXISTING KNOWLEDGE-BASE

Knowledge about coalitions is incomplete, at times conflicting, and lacks adequate connections between theory and practice. There are few systematic comparative studies of coalitions, and conceptual work has tended to be abstract and divorced from the real world. The few practice guides that exist seem elementary (Dluhy, 1981; Brown, 1984).

Conceptual work on coalitions has historically been found in the fields of social psychology, sociology, political science, and organizational development, and emphasizes game and decision theory, often utilizing experimental group data (Adrian & Press, 1968; Chertkoff, 1970; Caplow, 1968; Gamson, 1961; Komorita, 1978; Groennings, Kelley & Leiserson, 1970; Riker, 1962; Browne & Franklin, 1986; Gentry, 1987). Some writings on interorganizational work and networks are relevant to coalition-building (Strauss, 1978; Yanich, 1984; Rosenbloom, 1981; Karger & Reitmer, 1983; Aldrich, 1977; Boje & Wolfe, 1988; Agranoff & Lindsay, 1983; O'Toole & O'Toole, 1981; Whetten, 1981).

A spate of new literature on conflict resolution, negotiation, collaboration, and public-private partnerships, appealing to mediators, public administrators, and "community process workers" has contributed immeasurably to the knowledge of specific techniques (Carpenter & Kennedy, 1988; Gray, 1989; Fisher & Ury, 1981; Brooks, Liebman, & Schelling, 1984; Gricar & Brown, 1981; Moore, 1986; Raiffa, 1982; Susskind & Persico, 1983; Zartman & Berman, 1982). While some of this material can be applied to coalitions, much remains focused on more temporary and potentially adversarial parties that need to find agreement for purposes of mutual self-interest. Additionally, many of these sorts of collaborations are sparked by government or a private manager or mediator, and do not reflect self-forming, lasting coalitions.

Most community organizing textbooks and guides have paid minimal attention to the theory and practice of coalition-building (Brager, Specht, & Torczyner, 1987; Burghardt, 1983; Staples, 1984; Karger & Reitmeir, 1983; Cox et al., 1979; Kahn, 1982; Ecklein, 1984; Schwartz, 1965; Rubin & Rubin, 1986). Social workers have begun to describe and analyze coalition experiences and dynamics, but most work has been descriptive or anecdotal, using a case study approach or comparing a small number of coalitions (Black, 1983; Cromwell, Jr., Howe & O'Rear, 1988; Community Council, 1971; Pearl & Barr, 1976; Ortiz, 1981; Prigmore, 1974; Roberts-DeGennaro, 1986b; Weisner, 1983; Spiegel, 1981; Humphreys, 1979; Whitaker, 1982; Panet-Raymond, 1988; Ignacio, 1976). However, some integration of coalition theory and practice (Weisner, 1983; Roberts-DeGennero, 1986a, 1986b, 1987; Frey, 1974; Alicea, 1978) and substantive articles and books on coalitions are beginning to emerge in the applied social science and professional human service literature (Staggenborg, 1986; Kaplan, 1986; Downey, 1986; Sink & Stowers, 1989, Dluhy, 1990).

DEFINING SOCIAL CHANGE COALITIONS

Our research focuses on the social change coalition — which advocates for political, service, or other issues, in one or more arena ranging from neighborhood to international. This model has also been identified as "advocacy" (Dluhy, 1981; Roberts-DeGennaro, 1986a) "action" (Frey, 1974), "progressive" (Sink & Stower, 1989) and "grassroots" (Speigel, 1981).

Our working definition of the social change coalition is: a group of diverse organizational representatives who join forces to influence external institutions on one or more issues affecting their constituencies while maintaining their own autonomy. It is (a) an organization of organizations who share a common goal; (b) time limited; and (c) characterized by dynamic tensions.

METHODOLOGY

Our project expands the knowledge base of coalition-building by combining findings from the social science literature with practice wisdom. Based on our own experiences and an extensive literature review, we produced a background paper (Mizrahi & Rosenthal, 1986) which began to synthesize existing knowledge about coalitions and isolated key questions and conflicting information that needed further study. These unanswered questions were explored in a series of focus group seminars held by us in 1986-1988, in order to cull practice wisdom from coalition practitioners. In these sessions, participants explored their experiences in handling decisions critical to coalition development and endurance, and shared frustrations and successes. We also conducted a survey of 40 coalitions whose data are in the process of being analyzed.

The problems and solutions identified here are a composite of findings from the literature, as well as the collective experiences of over 50 coalition experts who shared their knowledge with us in these focus group seminars. The coalitions represented by these experts embraced four distinct types of goals and durations: *specific goal, short-term groups* (e.g., organizing demonstrations or forums), *specific goal, long-term* (e.g., banishing domestic violence, housing court reform); *general goal, short-term* (fighting crime or drugs), and *general goal, long-term* (neighborhood improvement coalitions, anti-racist networks).

The findings presented here are grouped within a framework we designed that isolates the dynamic tensions characteristic of coalitions. Examples of relevant approaches that have actually worked in practice are also presented to illustrate how certain dynamic tensions have been handled or avoided. Where there is related literature, it is cited.

THE COOPERATION-CONFLICT DYNAMIC

While shared goals and a willingness to work together are the foundation of coalition functioning, in fact social change coalitions are characterized by conflict as well as cooperation (Alicea, 1978). Conflict inherently occurs on several levels: (1) between the coalition and its social change target, around strategies and issues such as credibility, legitimacy, and power; (2) among the coalition participants around issues such as leadership, decision making, and personality/style; and (3) between the coalition and its member organizations around issues such as unshared goals, division of benefits, contributions, commitment, and representation.

Given these complex dynamics, coalition harmony cannot be sustained by appeals to rationality, facts, justice, and democratic process alone. Inherent conflict needs to be recognized and addressed creatively. Conflict is often expressed as opposition, disruption or impasse, or more covertly as passivity, inaction, withdrawal, and polite negativism. Since conflict is an inevitable part of the coalition dynamic, we maintain that coalition work should be approached as a conflict resolution model, where bargaining, trade-offs, negotiating, and compromise are part of all decisions, and agreements are reached by mutual consent (Strauss, 1978; Bacharach & Lawler, 1980; Levine, White, & Benjamin, 1961; Roberts-DeGennaro, 1987; Galeskiewicz, 1979; Cook, 1977). This is a fact well known by party or political coalitions. As mediating structures, coalitions must strive, not for unanimity, but for a way in which their members can work together (Miller, 1983). Maintaining flexibility around decision making and expectations for participation are essential. This may mean using methods of decision making that either allow for disagreement such as veto power or abstention, or require majority vote or consensus (Schwarz, 1970). Some groups further clarify what constitutes a majority as well as a critical number of dissenters (Downey, 1986). Coalitions can also provide a variety of ways for member organizations to express their involvement.

FOUR DYNAMIC TENSIONS

Arising out of this conflict/cooperation impulse are four dynamic tensions characteristic of coalitions. These are: (1) Mixed Loyalties; (2) Autonomy versus Accountability; (3) Means versus Models; and (4) Unity and Diversity.

1. *MIXED LOYALTIES: Coalition members have a dual commitment – to the coalition and to their own organizations, producing a conflict between altruism and self-interest.*

For those coalitions that operate in the same service or issue area as their member organizations, there may be competition for resources, as well as organizational time and energy, and confusion over which hat coalition members are wearing. Once a coalition is formed, this tension affects the degree of commitment and the contributions that members are willing to make to the coalition, as well as what the coalition can expect from them (Frey, 1974; Staggenborg, 1986).

Organizations frequently join coalitions for some protection, because they do not want to be visible on a particular issue. Yet, participating in a coalition means assuming a collective risk, presumably for a greater good or benefit. Both large, powerful organizations and small, struggling groups may decide not to join or to remain in a coalition because they want to control their own agenda, or because they are focused on their own survival (Groennings, 1970; Ortiz, 1981; Moberg, 1977; Caplow, 1968).

Coalitions have minimized losses and risks for member organizations by: (a) designing collective efforts that do not threaten the turf or networks or their member organizations; (b) identifying and treating carefully issues or positions that could compromise members' credibility and funding; (c) preventing direct competition between the member organizations and the coalition; and (d) agreeing on actions that organizations can do in the name of the coalition versus those that they do on their own.

> 2. *AUTONOMY V. ACCOUNTABILITY: The coalition must have enough autonomy to take independent action, and enough accountability to several levels within the coalition and its member organizations to retain credibility and maintain the base which is its essence.*

Effective coalitions eventually amass their own power and resources, and need to rely less upon their base (Gentry, 1987 quoting Hinkley). The intensity and urgency of interactions with the external target often demand swift, autonomous coalition action. Organizational representatives who cannot take independent action delay coalition response time (Zwier, 1987), and may, for this reason, be excluded from consistent involvement. As trust develops among active members, those who participate less frequently fall out of sync with the group's momentum. Experienced coalition-builders note lack of membership involvement as a major problem in sustaining participation (Roberts-DeGennaro, 1986b, Hartman, 1981; Kaplan, 1983; Weisner, 1983; Educational Priorities Panel, 1981; Clark, Martine, and Bartolomeo, 1988).

Appropriately involving each member organization is a time consuming but necessary task which can also slow the direct pursuit of social change goals. Coalitions have balanced the autonomy/accountability tension by creating a variety of ongoing communication mechanisms between the coalition and its members. They also clarify: how to integrate new members; whom the coalition represents; and when and how different levels of participants will be involved in coalition decisions and actions. Effective coalitions decide when they can assume or when they need to obtain sanction from the member organizations and their constituencies.

3. *MEANS V. MODEL: A coalition can be a means to accomplish a specific social change goal, as well as a particular model of sustained interorganizational coordination. Problems sometimes arise over which interpretation is to receive priority emphasis.*

Coalitions are usually viewed more as "means" than as "models" (Dhuly, 1981). Many groups could not visualize coalescing except when needed to reach specific social change goals. Only a few case studies depict coalitions as long-term "models," struggling with internal process and membership empowerment as goals (Downey, 1986; Roberts-DeGennero, 1986b; Harris, 1984; Kaplan, 1986; Schwarz, 1970). Experienced organizers and social critics now recognize the need to form long-term coalitions, moving more toward models than means (Kahn, 1982; Delgado, 1986; Miller & Tomaskovic-Devey, 1983).

Lack of clarity about whether the coalition is viewed primarily as a means or model can lead to differences in emphasis on process or product, degree of commitment, visions of success and failure, willingness to compromise, and time frame for accomplishment of coalition goal. People more concerned about results grow frustrated with lengthy decision-making processes and membership skills-building; people emphasizing the coalition as a model will sacrifice efficiency in order to strengthen internal development.

Coalitions primarily concerned about being a *model* emphasize: (a) a goal, structure and operating style that reinforces internal coalition development; (b) a commitment by member organizations to the coalition as an end in itself; (c) suspension of action toward the social change goal if necessary to build the coalition, itself. Some coalitions approached as a *model* later transform themselves into permanent organizations.

Coalitions primarily concerned about being a *means* to accomplish a specific goal: (a) provide "just enough" structure (Whitaker, 1982); (b) avoid time-consuming process issues; (c) promote involvement only to "produce results"; (d) either tolerate or find creative ways to work with differences. The most effective coalitions strive for consistency in process and goal, and balance skill and leadership development with coalition efficiency.

4. *UNITY AND DIVERSITY: Coalition members share compatible, but not identical, interests, and must both utilize diversity as a strength, and find ways to act in unison.*

Problems related to coalition unity/diversity can be found in the following eight dimensions: Goal; Ideology; Expected outcome; Power; Commitment; Contributions; Race, Sex, Sexual Preference, and Class; Organizational and Personal Styles. Due to this complexity, this article will concentrate on a more complete elaboration of the Unity/Diversity tension.

THE UNITY/DIVERSITY TENSION

Coalition members share compatible, but not identical, concerns. Consequently, they experience a simultaneous convergence and divergence of interests (Alicea, 1978). Coalitions need enough unity to act together and enough diversity to accomplish their goal and to represent a broad base. Their functioning requires a certain degree of "syncretism" — an attempt to combine or reconcile differing beliefs in all salient areas.

Coalition members must reach some amount of agreement regarding goals, strategies, domain, decision making, and evaluation (Benson et al., 1973). In the formative stage, the quest for unity compels many coalition leaders to recruit member groups of similar outlook or positive past alliances. Coalitions tend to form with familiar groups who share similar politics or religious ideology, locations in close proximity to each other, or past working relationships (Zwier, 1987; Browne & Franklin, 1986; Groennings, 1970). In so doing, they may exclude groups that could strengthen the coalition's credibility and impact on the social change target.

Many coalition leaders assume that unity demands uniformity and conformity. In fact, coalitions that are too unified resemble organizations, and fail to achieve the essence of the coalition — the inclusion of diversity. Moreover, excess unity can lead to competition among the groups for turf, access to resources or visibility (Roberts-DeGennaro, 1986b) and can also limit the coalition's creativity. Coalitions suffer if all their members have the same perspective, expertise, and resources: *In one case, womens' organizations coalesced to initiate statewide workplace fundraising to support their agencies, but as groups with similar resources and limited time, none could make the necessary commitment to see the project through* (Clark, Martine, & Bartolomeo, 1988).

Conversely, many coalitions pursue diversity, either strategically or indiscriminately. Clichés espousing this approach abound: "in numbers there is strength"; "the more the merrier"; "many hands make light work"; etc. In fact, numbers are not everything—rather, it is the specific mix of diversity needed for a "winning coalition" that is essential. Many groups leap over their differences initially, in pursuit of some common cause. Because people assume that working together will be easy, they may overlook differences that may impede coalition functioning over time (Kaplan, 1983; Harris, 1984; Renters' Alliance, 1980; Hartman, 1981).

Although there is an increasing recognition of the need to build diverse coalitions, especially across color and class lines, there are few documented analyses of effective intergroup efforts. Increasing a coalition's diversity will usually slow down progress toward external goals because it takes time to evolve trust, familiarity, and comfort (Reagon, 1983; Staggenborg, 1986; Carmichael & Hamilton, 1967).

Coalitions can become a whole that is greater than the sum of its parts, but to realize this great potential requires making creative use of the different components (Panet-Raymond, 1988; Kaplan, 1986): *A coalition for improved home care linked home care workers, unions, government agencies, and homebound clients around increasing the quality and monitoring of home care services and salaries of home care workers. An alternative budget coalition drew together a wide range of agencies receiving municipal funds in order to prevent the City from pitting one group against another.*

GOAL DIFFERENCES

Goal differences affect problem definition, identification of potential coalition members and choice of social change target, strategies, and solutions. Coalition participants may embrace the same general goal, but differ in its objectives.

When potential members cannot easily agree upon a common

goal, they tend to define goals either too narrowly or too broadly. A narrow goal may attract fewer adherents and consequently may limit a coalition's credibility or legitimacy: *A coalition advocating for broad housing court reforms would not espouse a specific single issue—a moratorium on evictions—which they considered to be tangential; those interested in that goal alone decided to form their own group.*

Conversely, a goal that is too broad may mislead participants, divert resources, and limit or lead to difficulty in selecting appropriate strategies: *One coalition's composition changed after they clarified that their goal "to improve the quality of life in a neighborhood" meant support for low-income housing rather than gentrification.*

It is best to define the goal broadly enough so that potential allies are not prematurely lost, but narrowly enough so that the coalition stands for something identifiable and can accomplish it. It is also important to refresh goals and objectives periodically. Goals change over time due to alterations in external conditions, as well as success or failure of the coalition's initial efforts. General goals such as peace, environmental protection, and ending poverty, take a long time to accomplish and require coalitions to build in interim milestones. Participants joining coalition efforts to achieve short-term victories need to be connected to the bigger picture; members committed to the long-term goal may need to build in additional incentives to ensure the sustained participation of others.

Managing Goal Differences

Coalitions utilize the following approaches to resolving or minimizing the problem of goal differences:

1. Select a goal that is central to everyone's interests and is seen as something that can benefit both the diverse groups and the coalition as a whole: *A highly diverse neighborhood improvement coalition advocated for economic development activities as well as mixed income housing that could benefit both low and middle income residents. A teen pregnancy coalition was able to include conservative church groups and pro-choice ac-*

tivists by defining their goals to include both prevention of teen pregnancy and assistance to teen parents.

2. Define a goal relevant to the members' interest, but broader than any one group could address alone: *A coalition of AIDS education and treatment programs worked together on a state comprehensive legislative agenda to fund a broad array of community-based services.*

3. Identify linkages between the issues: *A Latino-led coalition to oppose the "English Only" movement was able to attract participation from the Jewish community who could relate to this as a civil liberties issue.*

4. Create a superordinate goal that transcends differences among potential coalition members, and clarify how the participants' differences support the whole: *A housing advocacy coalition attracted participation from a wide range of housing, homeless, church and community groups because the policy it addressed — a formula for increased housing revenue — both superceded and directly affected the agenda of all its participants.*

5. Compromise on goals; create goals where all participants can get a portion of what they really want, enough to sustain their involvement: *An educational reform coalition maintained the involvement of special educators by modifying their goals for mainstream education to include the need for specialized Mental Retardation/Developmental Disabilities services outside the classroom.*

6. Change goals over time: *A coalition to fight the installation of a nuclear Navy port changed their action goals from mobilizing a voters' referendum (which failed) to successfully electing a mayor sympathetic to their cause.*

7. Show how short-term goals relate to the long term, bigger picture: *A coalition organized the largest anti-nuclear demonstration in history, as part of their long-term commitment to disarmament.*

IDEOLOGICAL DIFFERENCES

People with different political or religious ideologies approach coalition work with distinct belief systems and operating principles. The ideologies influencing coalition work may be a value-based commitment to a cause or a general concept of public interest. Organizations working within the same or different arenas may have conflicting ideologies on related issues: *Nuns and feminists may agree that battering women is unacceptable; coalescence is possible if they are willing to overlook each others' ideological differences on other issues (e.g., abortion).*

Ideologically-motivated groups have different incentives, energy to invest, and expectations about outcome than do groups who have joined a coalition for concrete results (Gamson, 1975). Both types of groups may fail to understand the worth of each other's concerns, injecting guilt and resentment into the mix. Groups with extreme ideologies find it more difficult to coalesce with others (Groennings, 1970; Staggenborg, 1986): *Black trade unionists in South Africa have worked with white corporate powers on economic development, although those committed to a Black liberation position would not do so. Sometimes ideology overshadows everything and makes collaboration impossible.*

Commonly, like ideologies are a compelling force for coalition formation (Zwier, 1987; Rapp, 1982). Ironically, ideologically similar organizations working in the same sphere often have greater difficulty working together—e.g., Communists and Socialists have difficulty forming lasting electoral coalitions—than do groups whose ideologies are farther apart. If the level of ideological disagreement is not as intense for one of the parties it will be easier for ideologically different groups to work together.

Managing Ideological Differences

Coalitions use the following approaches to help member groups with different ideologies work together more effectively:

1. Address a third issue unrelated to any member organization's domain: *Nationalist and integrationist African-American groups joined together when working on economic development for their communities.*

2. Take action only on issues on which there is total agreement and allow any group to have veto power (Schwarz, 1970).

3. Limit joint action strictly to goals: *Jewish groups joined Texas Oil Producers in a coalition to break the Arab oil cartel, which also had the effect of diminishing the power of the Arab states.*

4. Suspend judgment on areas of difference: *Gay rights groups and Catholic clergy have been able to work together on AIDS services and education.*

5. Compromise on public position: *Both pro-choice and anti-abortion groups worked well together in a coalition for peace once they agreed that neither group would have visible signs of their position on abortion at a public demonstration.*

6. Tone down the ideologically extreme position: *A Puerto Rican independence movement organization could work with more moderate Latino groups on civil rights, by holding their own ideology in check.*

DIFFERENCES IN EXPECTED OUTCOME

Organizations may agree on a common goal, but outcome expectations may differ if the goal directly affects their domain (Frey, 1974; Caplow, 1968). Ironically, the dilemma intensifies with a coalition's success, at which time decisions about pay-offs and rewards must be made.

Problems may emerge when the coalition decides how fought-for and won changes will be implemented: *Landlords and tenants had very different expectations about the outcome of working together on housing court reform, impeding agreement on candidate endorsement for judges. A nursing home coalition of consumers and providers agreed upon the need for greater reimbursement for ser-*

vices, but differed on how the additional funds obtained would be allocated.

When there is a zero-sum outcome, how to divide "the pie" (distributions and benefits) can become an issue: *A political coalition to defeat an incumbent mayor and to elect a minority candidate fell apart when its members could not agree on whether to run a Hispanic or an African-American candidate.*

Coalitions that form from a defensive or adversarial stance may have a problem developing a common proactive agenda. This is especially true when groups that fought for recognition by the social change target become recognized players or move from adversarial to advisory roles (Gamson, 1975; Sharp, 1981): *A number of groups who fought successfully against construction of a major highway had difficulty developing an alternative transportation plan.*

Coalitions can also offer variable sum, rather than zero-sum outcomes, where everyone may benefit. For example, political coalitions have recognized that influencing policy can be as important as controlling government offices (Reisinger, 1986). With multiple outcomes, however, there is a danger that the original goals can be diverted: *Different outcome expectations complicated the dynamics of a coalition of labor and welfare advocacy groups which formed to obtain a welfare grant increase. The unions were seeking support in the coalition for benefits for social service workers. The coalition fell apart when the union would not "sell out" its own constituency, and accepted the social change target's offer of concessions on worker issues without the increase in the welfare grant.*

Managing Outcome Expectation Differences

Coalitions withstand divergence in the outcome expectations of their members by the following means:

1. Expand or redefine the pie rather than consider possible outcomes in zero sum terms: *A local budget reform coalition of municipal grantees protested the City administration's determination to cut the City budget. Instead it created a proposal for alternative and increased revenues which would minimize service reductions.*

2. Engage on issues which promise some tangible or intangible gains for each coalition member (Reisinger, 1986): *A neighborhood-wide coalition formed in response to a needs assessment that indicated that the community was not receiving government or private funding proportionate to its problems. Participants determined that joint advocacy could bring in more resources to the community, which would be a tangible benefit to some, and an indirect benefit to all.*

3. Enable each member organization to maintain the ability to act autonomously on issues that are not directly related to coalition activity, and as long as they do not do so in the name of the coalition: *This is a policy of a coalition of Latino education advocacy groups who are all active on similar issues, join together on many larger fronts, but respect each other's individual priorities.*

4. Select coalition issues that do not conflict with members' individual agendas: *An educational reform coalition composed of advocacy and literacy groups, focused on reallocating the budget of the Board of Education, a task vital for all members, that did not compete with any one member's agenda.*

5. Make explicit the trade-offs for everyone's involvement: *Neighborhood groups approaching the same funding source agreed to advocate together for funds to create a joint homeless program, rather than secretly negotiating their own contracts.*

6. Discuss the consequences of winning or losing when there appears to be a zero sum outcome: *This applies to groups working for a candidate, a specific policy change, or a law.*

DIFFERENCES IN AMOUNT AND LEVEL OF POWER

Coalitions have to deal with the consequences of actual and perceived power differences among members and potential participants. Large powerful groups and institutions rarely join coalitions, because they have the necessary contacts, resources and constituencies to act independently. When powerful organizations do join coalitions it is usually for protection, legitimacy, and to reserve their resources for other interests (Staggenborg, 1986; Zwier, 1987; Hartman, 1979, 1981). Regardless of their direct actions, more powerful groups invoke among smaller organizations distrust, fear of cooptation, exploitation, and domination. Ironically, powerful groups are sometimes resented because others expect them to contribute more to a coalition than they actually do: *A national women's organization and several grassroots womens' groups joined forces on a womens' rights legislative initiative, but disparity in size and influence inserted distrust into their working relationship. In another case, power was actually exerted by an international union working in coalition with grassroots groups to organize an anti-apartheid demonstration. The union, which controlled most of the financial resources, imposed their management style on the coalition, alienating some of the grassroots participants.*

Managing Power Differences

To minimize power differences, coalitions find ways to have the powerful group provide resources without dominating. When it is desirable to keep the powerful group(s) inside the coalition, the following mechanisms may be established:

1. A one group/one vote rule (Stiles, 1988)
2. Voting/not voting membership
3. Caucuses for smaller groups
4. An agenda that gives less influential members the advantage: *One coalition changed from mainstream policy goals which benefited large agencies, to creation of a new government funding stream that gave awards to individual women who were leaders in less established settings.*

Coalitions which exclude powerful groups from full participation may continue to draw upon their resources and support by:

1. Making them affiliates or honorary members
2. Forming parallel/support coalitions (West, 1981)
3. Providing technical/advisory status for the powerful group.

DIFFERENCES IN LEVEL AND INTENSITY
OF COMMITMENT

Organizations join and continue participating in coalitions for a variety of pragmatic and/or ideological reasons. Pragmatic reasons include some degree of self-interest — a quest for resources, power or social contact; ideological motivations mean some shared value-based commitment to a cause or a concept of the "greater good."

Providing incentives for joining and sustaining coalition participation is critical (Zwier, 1987; Kaplan, 1986; Miller & Tomaskovic-Devey, 1983; Panet-Raymond, 1988; Roberts-DeGennaro, 1986b, 1987; Weisner, 1983; Staggenborg, 1986). Yet in practice, it is uncommon that coalition leadership and membership are conscious of their own expectations or responsibilities (Roberts-DeGennaro, 1986b).

Understanding the basis of commitment will reveal what is required to sustain it. The motivation for coalescing and the expectation of participation benefits should be fully explored, as should the source, amount, kind, and intensity of the member organizations' commitment. Misunderstandings and undue pressure may result because initial commitment as well as changes in commitment are rarely articulated.

Upon formation of a coalition, equal commitment is usually assumed, but in fact coalition work is always more important to some members than to others (Frey, 1974). Different levels of commitment result in differential readiness to act, take risks and responsibility, contribute resources, or represent the coalition (Rapp, 1982). Groups that view an issue as urgent or require the relationships offered by coalition participation will have a more intense commitment to coalition work. Some groups, sustained by their ideology, can devote more consistent energy to the coalition than can other groups. Over time, commitment to the coalition may change due to new factors operating inside the coalition, as well as changing circumstances affecting its members.

Differences in commitment also emerge when coalitions determine tactics and strategies: *A welfare advocacy coalition which included organizations funded by the City's welfare department as well as advocacy groups decided to negotiate rather than use militant tactics that would have compromised some of its members.*

Managing Differences in Commitment

To maximize commitment to the coalition effort and encourage a greater variety of organizations to participate, coalitions:

1. Structure opportunities for multiple levels of commitment: *One pro-choice lobbying coalition developed a three-tier system of participation, ranging from active lobbyists to information-seekers (Staggenborg, 1986).*

2. Develop membership agreements that clarify what kind and level of commitment is desirable and how it should be demonstrated: *One coalition insists that members make a half day a week commitment, to ensure that they are present at all meetings and involved in all decision making.*

3. Plan for fluctuations in commitment over time: *Many groups share or rotate leadership and arduous tasks.*

4. Provide a variety of incentives to sustain participation, addressing the actual motivations of members: *When members require results, coalitions have emphasized interim victories or redefined success in tangible terms. Some coalitions provide membership services, benefits and information. Others provide forums to enable participants to directly communicate and exchange their own expertise (Kaplan, 1986).*

5. Assure protection to members: *Some coalitions avoid compromising situations for their members by giving each member a chance to decide whether to take a publicly visible stance, or sign on to position papers or testimony.*

DIFFERENCES IN TYPE AND LEVEL OF CONTRIBUTIONS

The concept of pay-offs in exchange for members' contributions to the coalition was identified in the early experimental small group and game theory (Gamson, 1961), economic/cost-benefit models

(Riker, 1962), and in studies of political coalitions (Groennings, Kelley, & Leiserson, 1970). This literature emphasized the benefits of coalition participation, without paying enough attention to the costs (Adrian & Press, 1973).

The findings that not all coalitions win, that distributions of pay-offs vary, and that people will coalesce for reasons other than winning prompted many authors to review contextual environmental and situational elements of coalition participation (Browne & Franklin, 1986; Reisinger, 1986). The literature has begun to present a more balanced perspective on the trade-offs, pay-offs and exchanges needed to maintain effective coalitions (Weisner, 1983; Weiner, 1984; Panet-Raymond, 1988; Roberts-DeGennaro, 1986b).

Coalition development requires the assessment of the amount and kinds of contributions needed to form and maintain the coalition, and the assignment of equivalent weights to the various contributions actually provided by members. As coalitions endure, they identify whether they have the necessary contributions required both to achieve the social change goal and to maintain the coalition. If the mix is already correct, coalitions concentrate on sustaining these contributions. If it is insufficient on some dimension, a coalition will have to decide whether to compromise its position, settle for less, or change goals. Alternatively it could rearrange membership and/or contributions by increasing contributions from current members, replacing members who may have left, or expanding membership or recruiting more support from outside sources.

In practice, a variety of contributions are needed from participating organizations, dictated in part by goal, time and conditions. Yet, many coalitions do not clarify what constitutes a desirable or necessary contribution, or what the minimum contribution is. Participants have different expectations about what they can afford to contribute to the coalition and what they get back.

A problem arises because member organizations do not make identical contributions to the coalition. How should coalitions compare the worth of contributions such as: a powerful organization's name on a letterhead, a half day a week of volunteer time, a thousand signatures on a petition collected by a member? Contributions are differentially valued, and usually those members who contribute more gain greater control of the coalition and receive greater pay-offs.

Managing Differences in Contributions and Rewards

Effective coalitions clarify expectations about minimum contributions, how the ratio of contributions to rewards will be determined, and how differential contributions can be made to be equivalent. Some specific approaches include the following:

1. Balance contributions with rewards (Chertkoff, 1970; Gamson, 1961). There are several ways to do this:
   EQUITY: organizations get out what they put in.
   EQUALITY: regardless of what organizations put in, they get the same rewards.
   EQUIVALENCY (structured inequality): some organizations get out more than they put in, while others get less (Mizrahi & Rosenthal, 1986; Humphreys, 1979).

2. Determine minimum contributions according to a coalition's priorities: *One coalition decided to encourage members to contribute what they know and do best and as a result, contributions exceeded their expectations. Another one balanced its coalition needs for efficiency with members' desires to develop new skills.*

DIFFERENCES IN RACE, GENDER, SEXUAL PREFERENCE, AND CLASS

Longstanding differences in experiences, priorities, and problem definitions make it difficult to develop coalitions that cross race, gender, sexual preference, and class lines. Women and men appear to relate differently to coalitions and may have difficulty in working together (Caplow, 1968; Terhune, 1970; Gentry, 1987). Minority groups have many reasons to mistrust majority groups who have historically exploited, coopted, and dominated them. Arguments have been made against interracial coalitions (Carmichael & Hamilton, 1967; Marable, 1981; Eisinger, 1976). With few exceptions, even good faith efforts to sustain collaboration are impeded by this history (Reagon, 1983; Hartman, 1979, 1981; Harris, 1984).

Majority groups are accustomed to being in control, and are reluctant to give up power because in so doing, they also sacrifice a familiar way of working. As a result, minority group participants in diverse coalitions often risk the appearance or actuality of cooptation (Yanich, 1984). Soliciting minority participation is often perceived as tokenism, especially if it fails to cultivate or sustain meaningful involvement.

When minority individuals in majority dominated coalitions raise issues that are important to them, these are often dismissed as divisive: *A peace coalition with a significant lesbian and gay contingent disregarded feminist and gay issues and then fell apart because it never addressed the issues of greatest concern to significant numbers of their ranks.* On the other hand, majority groups often unfairly expect minority group members to assume the role of educator or conscience for the coalition, explaining or handling issues related to diversity.

Members of minority groups may have trouble coalescing with each other due to class, nationalist and gender divisions (Ortiz, 1981; Matloff, 1985; Gittell & Naples, 1982): *A Puerto Rican and African-American coalition for racial justice fell apart when it placed the legitimacy of one group above that of the other. Black women stopped working with men on Black nationalist goals in the 1960s because they felt their needs as women were disregarded. A coalition to pass the ERA found it difficult to sustain the participation of working class women's organizations.*

Managing Diversity in Race, Gender, Sexual Preference and Class

Coalitions consciously pursuing diversity factor in the time and effort to make it happen. Some effective efforts suggest the following:

1. Include diverse groups at the coalition's inception, rather than later, which can minimize real or perceived tokenism, paternalism and inequality.

2. Consciously give priority to increasing diversity: *One large coalition suspended work for three months on its goal to redevelop a huge waterfront parcel in order to recruit more poor people of color who lived in the area and would be directly affected by the project.*

3. A majority group-initiated coalition can offer some incentives ("affirmative action") to recruit minority participants, and consciously operate in new ways to share control and build trust. True diversity requires an ongoing commitment of coalition resources to issues of importance to the minority group members.

4. A minority group-initiated coalition can present its issues within a broad framework that integrates the majority perspective, if their involvement and support is deemed necessary.

DIFFERENCES IN ORGANIZATIONAL AND PERSONAL STYLE

Organizations and individuals bring different styles of operating and interacting to their coalition work. Organizational style differences are manifested in areas such as tolerance for conflict, decision-making and management methods, and expectations of organizational representatives and coalition leadership. Especially acute are style differences between political and human service organizations with respect to formality, process, strategies, and public stance (Frey, 1974; Weisner, 1983). Grassroots and professional groups have different skills in and reactions to written and verbal communication. They are comfortable in different arenas, and are often ignorant of the structure and culture of each other's organizations (Kaplan, 1983; Sampson, 1984; *Renters' Alliance,* 1980; Hartman, 1981). Sometimes different appearances reflect deeper organizational divisions which need to be acknowledged.

Some style differences evolve from race, class, and gender, and some, such as personality differences, are purely idiosyncratic (Terhune, 1970; Reisinger, 1986). Some people are comfortable talking a lot, while others prefer action. Some are boisterous at meetings, while others are listeners. However, sometimes what is perceived as a style difference in actuality masks a different ideology or agenda (Burghardt, 1983). It is important to analyze these style differences in order to understand whether they are dangerous or benign to coalition cohesion.

Managing Style Differences

Depending on their goal and the amount of time they have to act, coalitions either accept or attempt to minimize style differences. If there is a sense of urgency about taking coalition action, differences may be tolerated. Over the long term, coalitions committed to a model of intergroup cooperation have sought ways to minimize the negative effect of style differences. To contain differences which could become destructive, many coalitions spell out common rules for interaction:

1. Create and discuss ground rules for meetings and coalition operations.

2. Develop and enforce membership criteria.

3. Structure equal time to speak: *One coalition actually times speakers and asks everyone to say something or yield their turn to another.*

4. Conduct criticism/self-criticism of meetings which articulates and builds a common set of expectations, values and operating methods for coalition functioning.

5. Create a policy that allows for the exclusion of deviant or disruptive personalities or organizations, if necessary.

In each of the eight dimensions of the Unity/Diversity tension — goals; ideology; expected outcomes; power; commitment; contributions; race, gender, sexual preference, and class; and organizational and personal style — the challenge is to respect and plan for creative use of differences, as a way of building a unified coalition. Coalitions can be prepared for differences and provide a structure for member organization individuality, autonomy, dissent, and a productive synthesis of strengths.

CONCLUSION

Coalitions are complex organizations, born out of a desire or urgent need for intergroup action and cooperation. Coalitions must maintain unity while handling inevitable tensions that arise from their inherent diversity. Each of the eight dimensions of the unity/diversity tension described in this article are interactive, further complicating coalition dynamics.

Organizing and maintaining social change coalitions in the 1990s requires both an understanding of the theory underpinning such interorganizational entities and the application of the practice principles derived from collective experience. We suggest that curricula of professional schools, continuing education and staff development programs include such content. We also encourage collaboration between schools and agencies to conduct further grounded research for the purpose of synthesizing the theory and practice of coalition-building.

REFERENCES

Adrian, C.R. & Press, C. Decision costs in coalition formation. *American Political Science Review*, 1968, *62*, 556-563.

Agranoff, R. & Lindsay, V.A. Intergovernmental management: Perspectives from human services' problem solving at the local level. *Public Administration Review*, 1983, *43*, 227-237.

Aldrich, H. Visionaries and villains: The politics of designing interorganizational relations. *Organization and Administration*, 1977, *8*(2&3) 23-40.

Alicea, V.G. *Community participation, planning and influence: Toward a conceptual model of coalition planning*. Unpublished doctoral dissertation, Columbia University, 1978.

Bacharach, S.B. & Lawler, E.J. *Power and politics in Organizations*. San Francisco: Jossey-Bass, 1980.

Benson, J.K., Kunce, C.T., Allen, D. *Coordinating human services: A sociological study of an interorganizational network*. Columbia: University of Missouri, 1973.

Black, T.R. Coalition building: Some suggestions, *Child Welfare*, 1983, *62*, 263-268.

Boje, D.M. & Wolfe, T.J. Trans-organization development: Contributions to theory and practice. In H.J. Leavitt, L.R. Pondy, and D.M. Boje (Eds.), *Read-

ings in managerial psychology, (4th ed.). Chicago: University of Chicago, 1988.

Brager, G., Specht, H. & Torczuner, J.L. *Community Organizing* (2nd ed.). New York: Columbia University Press, 1987.

Brooks, H., Liebman, L. & Schelling, C. (Eds.) *Public-private partnership: New opportunities for meeting social needs.* Cambridge, MA: Ballinger, 1984.

Brown, C.R. *The art of coalition building: A guide for community leaders.* New York: The American Jewish Committee, 1984.

Browne, E.C. & Franklin, M.N. Editor's introduction: New directions in coalition research, *Legislative Studies Quarterly*, 1986, *11*, 469-483.

Burghardt, S. *Organizing for community action.* Beverly Hills, CA.: Sage, 1983.

Caplow, T. *Two against one: Coalition in triads.* Englewood Cliffs, NJ: Prentice Hall, 1968.

Carmichael, S. & Hamilton, C.V. *Black power: The politics of liberation in America.* New York: Vintage Books, 1967.

Carpenter, S.L., and Kennedy, W.J.D. *Managing public disputes: A practical guide to handling conflict and reaching agreements.* San Francisco: Jossey-Bass, 1988.

Chertkoff, J.M. Socio-psychological theories and research on coalition formation, in S. Groennings, E.W. Kelley & T.M. Leiserson, (Eds.) *The study of coalition behavior*, New York: Holt, Rinehart and Winston, 1970, 297-322.

Clark, Martine, & Bartolomeo, *The Womens' Funding Coalition: Why it did not succeed,* June 1988.

Community Council of Greater New York. *Report of the task force on recreational services for children and families on public assistance residing in hotels*, Summer 1971.

Cook, K.S. Exchange and power in networks of interorganizational relations. *Sociological Quarterly*, 1977, *18*,62-82.

Cox, F., Erlich, J., Rothman, J., & Tropman, J. (Eds.) *Strategies of community organization* (3rd ed.). Itasca, IL: F.E. Peacock Publishing Co., 1979.

Cromwell, H.S., Jr., Howe, J.W., & O'Rear, G. A citizen's coalition in mental health advocacy: The Maryland experience. *Hospital and Community Psychiatry*, 1988, *39*, 959-962.

Delgado, G. *Organizing the movement.* Philadelphia: Temple University Press, 1986.

Downey, G.L. Ideology and the clamshell and identity: Organizational dilemmas on the anti-nuclear power movement. *Social Problems*, 1986, *33*, 357-373.

Dluhy, M. *Changing the system: Political advocacy for the disadvantaged groups*, Beverly Hills, CA: Sage, 1981.

Dluhy, M.J., *Building Coalitions in the Human Services.* Newbury Park, CA: Sage, 1990.

Ecklein, J. *Community organizers* (2nd ed.). New York: Wiley, 1984.

Educational Priorities Panel. Building coalitions for educational priorities, New York City, June, 1981.

Eisinger, P.K. *The patterns of interracial politics: Conflict and cooperation in the city*. New York: Academic Press, 1976.

Fisher, R. & Ury, W. *Getting to yes: Negotiating agreement without giving in*. Boston: Houghton Mifflin, 1981.

Folberg, J., & Taylor, A. *Mediation: A comprehensive guide to resolving conflicts without litigation*. San Francisco: Jossey-Bass, 1984.

Frey, G. *Coalitions in community planning*. Unpublished doctoral dissertation, Brandeis University, 1974.

Galaskiewicz, J. *Exchange networks and community politics*. Beverly Hills, CA: Sage, 1979.

Gamson, W. *The strategy of social protest*, Homewood, IL: Dorsey Press, 1975.

Gamson, W. A theory of coalition formation. *American Sociological Review*, 1961, *26*, 373-82.

Gentry, M.E. Coalition formation and processes, *Social Work With Groups*, 1987, *10*, 39-54.

Gittell, M. & Naples, N. Activist women: Conflicting ideologies. *Social Policy*, 1982, *13*, 25-27.

Gray, Barbara. *Collaborating: Finding common ground for multi-party problems*. San Francisco: Jossey-Bass, 1989.

Gricar, B.G. & Brown, L.D. Conflict, power and organization in a changing community. *Human Relations*, 1981, *34*, 877-893.

Groennings, S. Notes toward theories of coalition behavior in multiparty systems: Formation and maintenance. In S. Groennings, et al. (Eds.), *The study of coalition behavior*. New York: Holt, Rinehart and Winston, 1970.

Harris, I. The citizens coalition of Milwaukee, *Social Policy*, 1984, *15*, 27-31.

Hartman, C. Running a rent control iniative campaign. *Shelterforce*, 1981, *6*, 6-7.

Hartman, C. Landlord money defeats rent control. *Shelterforce*, 1979, *5*, 3-5.

Humphreys, N.A. Competing for revenue-sharing funds. *Social Work*, 1979, *24*, 14-19.

Ignacio, L.F. The Pacific-Asian coalition: Origin, structure and program. *Social Casework*, 1976, *57*, 131-135.

Kadushin, C. Networking: No panacea, *Social Policy*, 1983, *13*, 45-48.

Kahn, S. *Organizing: A guide for grassroots leaders*. New York: McGraw Hill, 1982.

Kaplan, C. Class and coalition in New York City. *Social Policy*, 1983, *13*, 45-48.

Kaplan, M. Cooperation and coalition development among neighborhood organization: A case study. *Journal of Voluntary Action Research*, 1986, *15*, 23-34.

Karger, J.H. & Reitmeir, M.A. Community organization for the 1980s: Toward developing a new skills base within a political framework. *Social Development Issues*, 1983, *7*, 50-62.

Kelsey, J. & Wiener, D. Citizen/labor energy coalition. *Social Policy*, 1983, *13*, 15-24.

Komorita, S.S. Evaluating coalition theories, *Journal of Conflict Resolution*, 1978, *22*, 691-706.

Levine, S., & White, P. Exchange as a conceptual framework for the study of interorganizational relationships. *Administrative Science Quarterly*, 1961, *5*, 583-601.

Marable, M. Common program: a theoretical and historical critique on new strategies for black and progressive politics in contemporary America. *Catalyst*, 1981, *9-10*, 13-32.

Matloff, S. A practice-oriented bibliography on coalitions, with guide and working paper, Unpublished Paper, 1985.

Miller, S.M. Coalition etiquette: Ground rules for building unity. *Social Policy*, 1983, *14*, 47-49.

Miller, S.M. & Tomaskovic-Devey, D. A framework for new progressive coalitions. *Social Policy*, 1983, *13*, 8-14.

Mizrahi, T. & Rosenthal, B. Social change coalitions: Toward a synthesis of theory and practice, Unpublished paper, 1986.

Moberg, D. Chicago's organizers learn the lessons of CAP. *Working Papers for a New Society*, 1977, *5*, 14-19.

Moore, C. *The mediation process: Practical strategies for resolving conflict*. San Francisco: Jossey-Bass, 1986.

Ortiz, I.D. Chicano community organizations and the idea of ethnic coalitions: A case study. *Journal of Voluntary Action Research*, 1981, *10*, 85-98.

O'Toole, R., & O'Toole, A.W. Negotiating interorganizational orders. *Sociological Quarterly*, 1981, *22*, 29-41.

Panet-Raymond, J. A coalition for survival and initiative in changing times. Paper presented at Association for Community Organization and Social Administration, Seventh Annual Symposium, CSWE-APM, Atlanta, Georgia, March, 1988.

Pearl, G. & D.M. Barr. Agencies advocating together. *Social Casework*, 1976, *57*, 611-618.

Prigmore, C.S. Use of coalitions in legislative action. *Social Work*, 1974, *19*, 96-99.

Raiffa, H. *The art and science of negotiation*. Cambridge, MA: Harvard University Press, 1982.

Rapp, D.W. Ideology as an aspect of community organization and advocacy. *Social Development Issues*, 1982, *6*, 53-61.

Reagon, B.J. Coalition politics: Turning the century. In Barbara Smith (Ed.), *Home girls: Black Feminist Ideology*. New York: Kitchen Table Women of Color Press, 1983.

Reisinger, W.M. Situational and motivational assumptions in theories of coalition formation. *Legislative Studies Quarterly*, 1986, *11*, 551-563.

Renters' Alliance. San Francisco rent control: Analysis of a campaign. *Shelterforce*, 1980, *5*, 12-13.

Riker, W.H. *The theory of political coalitions*. New Haven: Yale University Press, 1962.

Roberts-Degennaro, M. Building coalitions for political advocacy efforts. *Social Work*, 1986a, *31*, 308-311.

Roberts-Degennaro, M. Factors contributing to coalition maintenance. *Journal of Sociology and Social Welfare*, 1986b, *13*, 248-264.

Roberts-Degennaro, M. Patterns of exchange relationships in building a coalition. *Administration in Social Work*, 1987, *11*, 59-67.

Rosenbloom, R.A. The neighborhood movement: Where has it come from? Where is it going? *Journal of Voluntary Action Research*, 1981, *10*, 4-26.

Rubin, H.J. & Rubin, I. *Community organizing and development*. Columbus, OH: Merrill, 1986.

Sampson, T. Coalitions and other relations. In L. Staples (Ed.). *Roots to power: A manual for grass roots organizers*. New York: Praeger, 1984.

Schwartz, M. Community organizing. *Encyclopedia of Social Work*, 1965. New York: National Association of Social Workers.

Schwarz, J.E. Maintaining coalitions: an analysis of the EEC with supporting evidence from the Austrian Grand Coalition: The CDU/CSW. In S. Groennings, E.W. Kelley & M. Leiserson, (Eds.). *The study of coalition behavior*. New York: Holt, Rinehart and Winston, 1970.

Sharp, E. Organizations, their environments and goal definition: An approach to the study of neighborhood associations in urban politics. *Urban Life*, 1981, *9*, 415-439.

Sink, D.W. & Stowers, G. Coalitions and their effect on the urban policy agenda. *Administration in Social Work*, 1989, *13*, 83-89.

Speigel, H.B.C. Coalitions of grass roots groups. *Citizen Participation*, March/April, 1981, *4*, 8.

Staggenborg, S. Coalition work in the pro-choice movement: Organizational and environmental opportunities and obstacles. *Social Problems*, 1986, *5*, 374-390.

Staples, L. *Roots to power: A manual for grassroots organizers*. New York: Praeger, 1984.

Stiles, G.M. What makes a coalition successful. Paper presented at a Leadership Conference for Health Care Contributors. Chicago, September, 1988.

Stoner, M. R. Building local coalitions against the conservative tide. *Social Welfare Forum*, 1982-83. Washington: National Conference on Social Welfare, 1985.

Strauss, A. *Negotiations*. San Francisco: Jossey-Bass, 1978.

Susskind, L. & Persico, S. *Guide to consensus development and dispute resolution techniques*. Cambridge, MA: Harvard Negotiation Project, 1983.

Terhune, K.W. The effects of personality in cooperation and conflict. In P. Swingle (Ed.), *The structure of conflict*. New York: Academic Press, 1970.

Weiner, H. Survival through coalitions. In F. Perlmutter (Ed.), *Human services at risk*. Lexington, KY.: D.C. Heath, 1984.

Weisner, S. Fighting back: A critical analysis of coalition building in the human services. *Social Service Review*, 1983, *57*, 291-305.

West, G. *The national welfare rights movement: The social protest of poor women.* New York: Praeger, 1981.

Whetten, D.A. Interorganizational relations: a review of the field. *Journal of Higher Education*, 1981, *52*, 1-28.

Whitaker, W.H. Organizing social action coalitions. In M. Mahaffey and J.W. Hands (Eds.). *Practical politics and political responsibility.* Washington, D.C.: NASW, 1982.

Yanich, B. Urban community partnerships: Symbols that succeed and strategies that fail. *Journal of Voluntary Action Research*, 1984, *13*, 23-37.

Zartman, W. & Berman, M. *The practical negotiation.* New Haven: Yale University Press, 1982.

Zwier, R. Coalition strategies of religious interest groups. Paper presented at American Political Science Association Meeting, September, 1987.

Nurturing Grassroots Initiatives for Community Development: The Role of Enabling Systems

David M. Chavis, PhD
Paul Florin, PhD
Michael R. J. Felix, BA

There is a rapidly developing realization that the co-production of services by citizens and community institutions is essential for positive and sustained change to occur (Rich, 1979; Spiegel, 1987). Community participation, largely through the efforts of voluntary associations, has been advocated in the areas of urban service delivery (Rich, 1979); health promotion and disease prevention (Green, 1986); crime and drug abuse prevention (Curtis, 1987); welfare reform (Moynihan, 1986); and mental health service delivery (Naparstek, Beigal, & Spiro, 1982). Changes in health promotion strategies reflect larger domestic and international trends toward decentralization and participatory democracy.

Policies that intended to mobilize "the community" to address social problems have been used before (i.e., the Model Cities Program). It would be wise to approach the current situation with wisdom gained from these earlier efforts. The most common criticisms

Dr. Chavis is Associate Director, Center for Community Education, School of Social Work, Rutgers University, 73 Easton Avenue, New Brunswick, NJ 08903. Dr. Florin is Associate Professor, Psychology Department, University of Rhode Island, Kingston, RI 02881. Mr. Felix is a private consultant, 1455 F Street, Suite 250, N.W. Washington, DC 20005.

This study was funded in part by the Kaiser Foundation. The authors express appreciation also to J.R. Newbrough, Lawrence Green, Terry Mizrahi, and John Morrison for their comments on earlier drafts of this paper.

of the War on Poverty during the 1960s in the United States include the following: little, if any, implementation of comprehensive planning; a limited support system for community programs; the establishment of a new system which by-passed local authorities and other "powers" in the community; insufficient local coordination across sectors and among government agencies; and insufficient funding, in part due to dependence on federal rather than local sources; and an absence of any examination of what was available locally. (Moynihan, 1969; Washnis, 1974).

This article advocates the development of a support system for community organization and development or an "enabling system" that can address two central challenges facing those who would employ grassroots community initiatives as a central mechanism for tackling entrenched social problems and promoting social change. The first challenge involves the organizational vulnerability of voluntary community organizations. Despite the variety of positive impacts produced by voluntary community organizations, they are vulnerable to rapid decline or dissolution. Research has found that voluntary community organizations have high rates of "mortality" or at least inactivity (i.e., they stop meeting, become disorganized). Fifty percent of voluntary neighborhood associations were found to become inactive after their first year (Prestby & Wandersman, 1985; Yates, 1973). The maintenance of voluntary community organizations is a greater challenge in many ways than their formation. We know relatively little about what can be done to help voluntary community organizations survive and become more effective.

The second challenge involves efficiently and effectively supporting large numbers of voluntary community organizations. Thousands of voluntary community organizations already exist across the nation (Florin, 1989). If ambitious goals such as significant increases in health or decreases in substance abuse or crime are to be reached by employing voluntary community organizations and other institutions, additional thousands will need to be created. Developing "demonstration" programs in only one or a few communities at a time is insufficient. The time lapse for demonstrations to be documented and disseminated to other communities is too long, while problem situations remain unaddressed and rampant in most communities. Furthermore, the standard practice of supporting voluntary community organizations through individual case consultation or staff intensive methods can't meet the challenge because resources and trained personnel are limited. An approach must be developed which can deliver resources and incentives that increase the problem solving capacity of communities, largely through voluntary community organizations, to manage and control change on a sustained basis.

An analogy can be drawn from common sense practices in the field of agriculture: A farmer who tries to cultivate each plant on his or her plot on an individual basis will soon exhaust his or her capabilities; rather, the farmer is well advised to apply "enabling systems" such as tilling, seeding, irrigation and hoeing across the entire field. The challenge therefore, is to create the fertile and healthy environment within which many organized community initiatives can grow and be nurtured.

We see these two challenges as crucial for the advancement of "community" approaches to social problem solving by social workers and other health and human services planners. Currently, there is neither an accepted "social technology" nor sufficient research on capacity building and support systems available for community organizations. We believe that systems concepts can help us meet both challenges.

THEORETICAL AND RESEARCH CONTRIBUTIONS TO UNDERSTANDING HOW TO SUPPORT COMMUNITY INITIATIVES

A number of theories and research efforts can assist us in developing the technology to address the challenges of supporting the development, maintenance, and growth of large numbers of community organizations. Relevant theories include general and open systems theory, network theory, social learning theory, adult education, and behavior theory. An understanding of these theories will aid the human services planner and other practitioners in designing the support system for community based and community development initiatives.

General systems theory (Berrien, 1968; von Bertalanffy, 1950) has been applied to human social organizations (Katz & Kahn,

1978; Murrel, 1973; Plas, 1986). Open systems theory (Katz & Kahn, 1978), a specific application of general systems theory, assists us in understanding what it takes for organizations to develop, maintain themselves and grow by examining the flow of resources or energy.

The basic open systems concept, applied to voluntary community organizations (e.g., coalitions, neighborhood associations, self-help groups), is that the community organization receives various *input* from its environment (e.g., information, potential members, money). Input is transformed within the organization and becomes *throughput*. Within the throughput there are structures and functions performed by the organization that constitute subsystems with the purpose of using energy or resources to either maintain the organization (i.e., making sure the organization remains viable) or produce the intended goals of the organization (e.g., improving the quality of life for community members).

Organizational activities result in intended and unintended outcomes, or *output* in turn upon leaving the organization. Outputs become part of the environment, which in turn sends feedback (an input) back to the organization. Figure 1 illustrates this model as it has been applied to voluntary community organizations (Florin et al., in press).

Community organizations, like all systems, have forces that rush toward disorganization and "death" (entropy). To survive, community organizations must counter this process through "negative entropy" — importing more energy from the environment than they will use. A system will first spend its energy collecting inputs or resources, later transforming them for the maintenance of the organization and then for production. Community organizations expend high levels of energy collecting inputs (recruiting members, raising money) and transforming them into throughput (activities and programs). These organizations must build a highly efficient capacity to gain access to and use resources in order to survive.

Community organizations must be capable of regularly receiving information on their environments such as assessing community needs and strengths. Negative feedback — criticism from the community, a failed project — allows the system to make adjustments to enhance its ability to maintain itself. Voluntary community organi-

Figure 1: A SYSTEMS FRAMEWORK

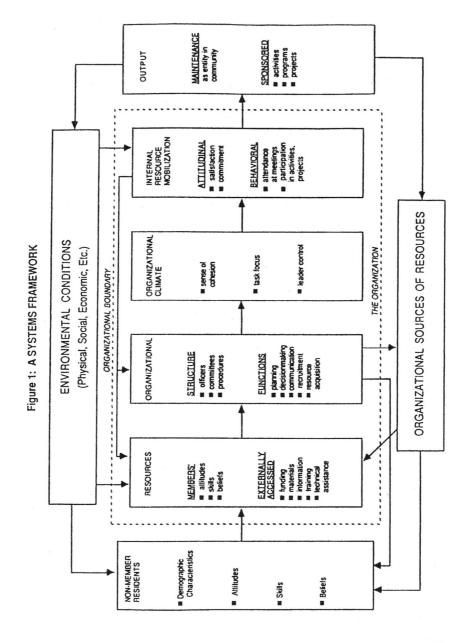

45

zations require information (inputs) concerning the resources in their environment (e.g., grants, technical assistance, other groups they could work with, innovations) and their immediate environment's conditions (e.g., community needs and information on competing systems).

The organization also needs information about its own internal functioning in order to make appropriate adjustments, just as people need to know their body temperature, weight, blood pressure, etc. Key indicators need to be identified (e.g., needs of members, available funds), and regular monitoring is necessary. Survey-guided feedback methods on key components of the organization's internal functioning have been found to reduce the rate that organizations become inactive by 50 percent (Chavis & Florin, 1990).

Theories of networks, social learning and adult education provide knowledge that can be useful for addressing the needs of community organizations identified by general systems theory. All of these theories have had substantial empirical and experiential validation.

Networks are interconnected and interactive social relations among various nodes or points. A node can be an individual person or an organization. Fischer (1977) has described networks as "a specified set of links among social actors." Network analysis provides a paradigm to examine networks. The structure of the network can also be examined in terms of its density (frequency and completeness of interaction) and its components (e.g., nodes, linkages, brokers).

Network theory also examines the flow of resources. A network can be defined by the recipients involved in transactions where common resources are exchanged (Cook, 1982). Reciprocity is important to the network in order to maintain its balance. The transactions within the network are often indirect and not always mutual (Levi-Strauss, 1969). The network, therefore, needs to encourage within itself as many combinations of exchanges as possible. There is also a norm or a mutually held expectation of reciprocity that overshadows all relations, among individuals and organizations, within the network (Gouldner, 1960). An important strategy for the enabling system is to provide many sustained and unrestricted opportunities for exchange, sharing, or interaction among all participants (e.g., community organizations, technical assistance providers, government agencies at all levels, etc.).

The distribution of resources within a network is controlled by "brokers." Brokers develop power, and the network becomes dependent on them regardless of their intentions (Marsden, 1982). Dependency is created as a function of the broker's role and behavior. The different providers of support in an enabling system are brokers. It is recommended that within the enabling system there be decentralization of the brokering role and behaviors. Mechanisms for maintaining the accountability of the system should also be considered (e.g., governmental oversight, citizen participation in monitoring, a mandatory majority consumer representation in the governance of the system).

Network density is another important consideration for the design of an enabling system. Density is determined by the number of lines of exchange or communication within the network. Dense networks frequently exchange among themselves; there is greater overlap among exchanges, and they rarely exchange outside their networks. A cohesive ethnic community would be considered a dense network. Members of less dense networks or ones with "weak ties" (Granovetter, 1973) exchange as much or more outside the network. Cohesive and dense networks provide greater support for its members and rapid communication. According to Granovetter (1982), weak ties have been found to be more conducive to the transfer of cultural and other innovations and they provide greater potential for collaboration. An enabling system needs to balance the strengths of ties among its members. It appears to be essential to keep the network open to exchanges with other networks, to interact and incorporate other social policy areas, to involve interdisciplinary actors, and to limit the sense of community among its members.

Social learning theory (Bandura, 1986; Parcel, Taylor, Brink, Gottlieb, Engquist, O'Hara & Erickson, 1989) and theories of adult education (Freire, 1970; 1985; Knowles, 1970; 1978; Knox, 1986) offer the enabling system strategies for building the capacity of local communities through the education and development of citizens. The services offered through the enabling system according to these theories, should: be problem oriented; be experiential learning, based on simulations and actual real life-experiences; be directed by the learner and his/her needs; allow for different learning styles; be sustained and readily accessible as questions and barriers emerge; use role modeling and peer learning (learning from people like oneself); be proactive; offer on-going support to participants; use multiple, mutually reinforcing methods; provide incentives for participation; and promote the adoption of new ideas.

Social scientists have begun to document the effectiveness of methods based on these theories for supporting community development corporations (Vidal, Howitt & Foster, 1986), voluntary community organizations and other neighborhood associations (Chavis & Florin, 1990; Speigel, 1987) health promotion programs (Merino, Fisher & Bosch, 1985) and self-help groups (Bernstein, in press; Julien, 1988; Madera, 1986; Maton, Leventhal, Madera & Julien, 1989).

These theories and research findings serve as the foundation for our description and recommendations for the development of enabling systems.

ENABLING SYSTEMS

An enabling system is a coordinated network of organizations which nurtures the development and maintenance of a grassroots community development process through the provision of resources, incentives and education. The goal of an enabling system is to support sustained community problem solving and development. Enabling systems consist of intermediary support organizations and resource networks that broker resources from larger systems for use by community organizations. Intermediary support organizations can include technical assistance and consultation services. Technical assistance services focus primarily on activities that address a social problem (e.g., drug-abuse prevention) or a common organizational need (e.g., nonprofit management). The resource network can include a variety of other organizations which address the production (social problems) or maintenance (organizational) needs of their client organizations. Together, intermediary support organizations and resource networks provide systemic supports such as conferences, workshops, recognition events and other activities to be discussed later in this paper.

Another defining characteristic of an enabling system is operations across different geographic levels. Local structures of the system (e.g., voluntary community organizations; city-wide coalitions) increase the psychological and physical accessibility of the system to the communities and provide more efficiently sustained assistance. Larger structures (e.g., a county wide, state or national network) allow for better dissemination of innovation and knowledge. Larger systems can also more economically produce resources (e.g., publications, planning tools, curriculum, media) that address common needs among many organizations at the local level.

Examples of Enabling Systems

Enabling systems of broad but varying scope exist within the United States forming linkages to hundreds or thousands of grassroots organizations. They qualify as self-contained enabling systems because of their breadth of operations and multiplicity of services, and specificity of problems to solved. The following are some examples:

The United Way of America, located in Alexandria, VA, supports over 2,300 locally controlled United Way organizations throughout the U.S. They provide staff and volunteer training, prepackaged materials or tools for fundraising, community problem planning and management, conferences, publications, and other services.

The *Citizens Committee for New York City* annually assists 3,000 volunteer-based neighborhood organizations (e.g., block and tenant organizations) and maintains contact with about 10,000 groups. Leadership and organizing training, technical assistance in crime and drug-abuse prevention, publications, coalition development, seed or incentive grants, and awards are among the many services they provide.

The *cooperative and agricultural extension services* have been in existence since 1908 to help rural America achieve social and economic stability through technology transfer and community development. These programs generally are operated through state universities and colleges with offices in each county within the state. Assistance, primarily in rural areas, is provided in regard to agriculture, family issues, health, and community development.

The *Neighborhood Reinvestment Corporation* provides assistance to neighborhood housing development and rehabilitation programs in 165 cities throughout the U.S. The local organizations represent a partnership of neighborhood residents, businesspersons and government representatives. Through a combination of state, regional and national field service centers, support is lent to organizational and community development needs while disseminating technical knowledge of finance and home construction or rehabilitation.

There are 27 states with *self-help clearinghouses*. The most extensive systems exist in California, Illinois, New Jersey, and New York. Their primary function is to connect citizens with self-help groups. Almost all of the clearinghouses provide assistance in the development and maintenance of self-help groups including workshops, conferences and publications. The New Jersey Self-Help Clearinghouse, for example, has aided in the development of over 500 self-help groups over the last eight years. State and local clearinghouses interact through the International Network of Mutual Aid Centers. Research and evaluation have been relatively well-integrated into the national and some of the state systems.

STRUCTURES AND ELEMENTS OF ENABLING SYSTEMS

Enabling systems that effectively and efficiently stimulate community initiatives and development require specific structures and program elements. Enabling systems that have been put into practice (such as the previous examples) generally use *resource networks* and *intermediary support organizations* as the main vehicles to deliver their services.

A *resource network* "maximizes mutual support and the exchange or resources" (Sarason, Carroll, Maton, Cohen, & Lorentz, 1977). It is "a type of network sustained not only because it increases resources available to people or expands their knowledge, or provides new experience, but also because it dilutes the sense of loneliness" (Sarason et al., 1977). Resource networks provide linkages between intermediary support organizations and community organizations. These are horizontal organizations (Robinson, 1986); the exchange of resources and decision making is collaborative. Network exchanges also are provided regularly among support organizations (e.g., technical assistance organizations) and community organizations.

Intermediary support organizations play a central role in an enabling system. They broker and transform resources from larger or different systems for use by more local organizations. They implement the functions of the enabling system through their services. There can be one or more intermediary support organizations in an enabling system. Examples of intermediary support organizations are: technical assistance organizations, information clearinghouses, consulting organizations, training centers, research organizations, voluntary action centers, and media and marketing organizations. There are also multi-faceted organizations that include all or almost all of the elements of an enabling system such as the Local Initiatives Support Corporation, Enterprise Foundation, Center for Community Change, Health Promotion Resource Centers, National Crime Prevention Council, United Way of America, units of government, university-based programs and others mentioned in this paper. Chavis (1990) has identified over 600 of these organizations in the U.S.

Multiple Community Sites: Multiple community sites, even within the same city or county are serviced by an enabling system. These multiple sites may be composed of community organizations, task forces, coalitions, or other "community" entities. Multiple sites are necessary for a number of reasons: the content task of some enabling systems (e.g., health promotion, substance abuse prevention) requires the mobilization of many sites and institutions; multiple sites provide a mechanism for reaching further into the grassroots; multiple sites can support each other and exchange ideas with each other; and certain "economies of scale" exist for performing some enabling system functions (e.g., costs for preparing and publishing a resource directory may be similar for 20 or 100 copies).

Incubators. Innovative and entrepreneurial ventures need opportunities to grow at the grassroots level. This element is closely related to supporting multiple community sites because more program variety and innovation can be "incubated" in many sites simultaneously than in one or two demonstration sites. Neighborhood Reinvestment, for example, encourages local programs to develop new programs to respond to the conditions in participating communities by providing seed capital and technical assistance.

Seed Capital and Incentives. Mobilization of community sites and stimulation of innovative programs can be sparked through incentive grants which provide seed capital and through incentives such as awards and the publicity which recognizes successful community efforts. The Citizens Committee for New York City (CCNYC) provides an excellent example of this process. CCNYC solicits funds from a variety of public and private sources. It then distributes them in the form of small incentive and seed grants of $50 to $3,000. These grants, combined with a program that recognizes model programs and technical assistance, is strategically designed to foster innovation and encourage community groups to move into new areas of problem solving or organizational development. Generally all applicants either receive a grant or some other form of recognition — everyone wins.

Multi-Sectoral Collaborative Structures. If broad-based solutions are to engage a variety of local resources, representatives from all sectors of the relevant community sites must be brought together in joint community problem solving. These types of "partnerships" or coalitions involve such sectors such as government, business, colleges and universities, health and human service providers, leaders of the powerful and relatively powerless, schools, and churches. The Georgia Planning Group for Health Promotion is made up of the leadership of the Georgia Missionary Baptist Convention, the State Department of Health, Voluntary Healthy Agencies and the Morehouse School of Medicine. The purpose of this group is to foster a partnership among the African-American churches, the local health departments, and other community resources in 27 rural communities in order to more effectively address drug abuse, heart disease, and adolescent pregnancy.

Multi-sectoral involvement enables the development of comprehensive solutions to complex social problems. This type of strategy is currently being implemented in the state of Mississippi whereby an enabling system will be developed through the Governor's office directly to support initiatives at the grassroots level by combining resources at the State and local levels in the areas of health, housing, economic development, education, and social services. This approach will include coalitions at the state and local level as well as with a primary reliance on voluntary community participation and organization.

FUNCTIONS OF AN ENABLING SYSTEM FOR COMMUNITY DEVELOPMENT

An enabling system may contain a very wide variety of service or functions. Table 1 summarizes these services and identifies the organizational target and whether the service is assumed to have a direct or indirect effect on the individual within the organization, the organization as a whole, the immediate target community or larger service/political (macro) systems. Table 1 can be used as an aid to planning support services within an enabling system. Particular services can be delegated among multiple intermediary support organizations where they exist or where resources are limited strategies with the most impact on the problem situation can be chosen. In this way strategic planning can allow for the greatest number of communities to be served with limited resources.

The specific functions of the enabling system, provided through the services of intermediary support organizations and resource networks, are targeted at capacity building throughout the multiple community sites. Garkovich (1989) has stated that "if community development as a discipline and a practice is to be relevant to the needs of the communities of tomorrow, the challenge is to shift the focus of training and activities to the more difficult and time-consuming, yet eminently more effective, strategy of local capacity building" (p. 215). We define community capacity as the ability of a community to mobilize and use resources for problem solving and development. Three general types of strategies for community capacity building have been identified and the functions of the enabling system address all three.

Table 1

CORE SERVICES WITHIN AN ENABLING SYSTEM

AND THEIR IMPACT

SERVICES:	INDIVIDUAL WITHIN THE ORGANIZATION	THE ORGANIZATION	LOCAL COMMUNITY	MACRO SYSTEM
Training	X	O		
Publications	X	O		
Communication/Public Education	X	X	X	X
Consultation with Staff and Leaders	X	O		
Organizational Development, Team Training and Consultation	X	X	O	
Rewards and Recognition	O	X	O	O
Advocacy and Empowerment	O	O	X	X
Networking and Coalition Building	X	X	O	X
Needs Assessment/Problem Solving	X	X	X	X
Collecting and Distributing Resources	X	X	X	X
Information and Referral/Linkages	X	X	X	X
Research & Development/Evaluation	X	X	X	X
Marketing	X	X	X	X
Generating Vision	X	X	X	X

DIRECT EFFECT= X
INDIRECT EFFECT=O

Expanding the Base of Citizen Involvement

An enabling system expands the base of citizen involvement through networking, promoting collaboration, and developing community ownership:

Networking. Resource exchange networks among community organizations can be developed around common problems and/or common geographic areas. It has been our experience that the exchange periods have been the most favorably rated part of training program. Intermediary support organizations can encourage resource-exchange networks by supporting meetings of network members and providing assistance in the facilitation of these meetings. Newsletters have been useful in the maintenance of resource exchanges between meetings (Robinson, 1986).

Promoting Collaboration. Collaborative structures such as coalitions and partnerships need to be cultivated in order to foster ownership and maximize the use of community resources. Intermediary support organizations can convene such groups. They also can provide situations where those type of groups can be developed.

Development of Community Ownership of Problem Solving. This function is fulfilled in two ways. The first is to ensure that local communities have the capacity to assess their needs and strengths and to develop strategies that gain widespread support. Included in this process is the assurance that the local community will have long-term support from both internal and external resources. It is also essential that disenfranchised and at-risk groups be included. The second is through the decentralization of the enabling system and the development and maintenance of local intermediary support organization, that are preferably (if not ultimately) within each community.

Enhancing the Leadership Pool and Augmenting Leadership Skills

An enabling system enhances the leadership pool available in a community and augments leadership skills through direct training for leadership, team-training methods and organizational development techniques:

Leadership Training: A major service is leadership skills training (e.g., advocacy, planning, meeting management, delegation, negotiation) and other forms of adult education including the training of staff and volunteers to perform vital community development and problem-solving activities.

Team Training: Team-training methods involve the development of a core group to operate collectively within a community site. This strategy has a number of advantages over training individuals. The most basic is that the responsibility for transferring the acquired knowledge back to the community or organization is shared, and training program objectives are more likely to be accomplished. Team training also allows workshops to be more relevant to the participants' situation, because teams can spend time on activities that are relevant to their own situation. This results in a greater likelihood that plans developed at a workshop will be implemented. Team training can be considered an intervention with a higher "dosage strength" than traditional individual training designs.

Organizational Development Techniques: Organizational development techniques such as team building, participatory strategic planning, and group problem-solving are another group of services that support the leadership enhancement function of the enabling system. These services are more labor intensive and require a greater variety of skills and experience on the part of the provider. They also have a greater effect on the organization and its community than training methods alone.

A critical challenge for this group of services is to provide sustained support. There needs to be active follow-up to training workshops and organizational development activities. Telephone contact following a workshop may be all that is needed in some cases. Other follow-up activities, such as informal meetings between workshop participants, should also be considered.

Expanding the Information and Resource Base

An enabling system expands the information and resource base available to community sites by brokering resources and information, dissemination and diffusion of models, promoting experimentation, and research and development.

Brokering of Resources and Information. The most basic function of an enabling system that intermediary support organizations can provide is the direct provision of information and resources or referral to other appropriate resources. It is not necessary for the intermediary support organization to itself contain all the knowledge or expertise to address every possible situation or need of their constituency community sites. It is essential, however, that there be knowledge within the system of where those resources exist and ability to provide adequate referral which includes monitoring, evaluation, and follow-through.

Financial resources can also be distributed through intermediary support organizations. Grants, loans and other financial resources can be obtained from governments, foundations, and corporations and distributed to the community sites serviced by the intermediary support organizations on competitive and non-competitive bases. The intermediary support organizations allow financial allocations easy access to community organizations, due to their established networks and low overhead. Network members are involved in the distribution of the resources.

Dissemination and Diffusion of Models. The distribution of printed descriptions of model programs through publications or newsletters expose community leaders and planners to new ideas for potential adoption. Pipelines to potential solutions from outside the local geographical area therefore need to be established. Presentations, videos and site visits can lead to effective adoption (Parcel et al., 1989) but the intent to adopt a successful program must be supported with appropriate capacity development and adaptation to local conditions. If, however, the community and key influentials within it have not developed ownership of the problem and the solution and do not see a valuable role for themselves to play, the likelihood of adoption is slight regardless of support services (Rodgers, 1983; Rothman, 1980). Generic models of problem solving or conflict resolution strategies are best assimilated through experiential learning formats which permit practice and practical application the variety of situations most encountered by the participants.

Experimentation. The enabling system functions to support local experimentation through the use of seed grants to multiple community sites and its research and development services. The multiple community sites are all considered incubators of innovations as local experimentation is a general function pervading the system rather than one confined to a few particular demonstration or research sites. Locally grown solutions are systematically examined and distilled for successful or promising approaches which can be replicated in other sites.

Research and Development. The enabling system should be guided by information on the environment as well as information that improves our knowledge of the issues being addressed and the methods used to address them. The goal is to have an intelligent system — one capable of learning, growing, and adapting. Research and evaluation services should be integrated into the enabling system as part of an intermediary support organization, rather than a function that is provided outside of the system. Program audits, requiring an independent evaluator, can be appropriate at times. However, in order to provide the most efficient and effective informational inputs for the proper functioning of the system, this function needs to come from within the system. Research and evaluation efforts that are initiated by intermediary support organizations in collaboration with their network members are less likely to be met with resistance from participants and the products are more likely to be useful and "owned" by members of the system.

The research and development function goes beyond evaluation, environmental monitoring, and market research. Intermediary support organizations provide an ideal setting for the development of social technologies that address community problems or improve community initiative, viability, and maintenance. Methods for social technology have been developed (Fawcett, Seekins, Whang, Muiv & Suarez de Balcazar, 1984; Rothman, 1980), but the setting that offers the opportunity for research and technology development along with technology transfer has not been clearly identified (Varela, 1970). Intermediary support organizations can provide the opportunity for technology development, transfer and diffusion.

PRINCIPLES FOR THE OPERATION
OF AN ENABLING SYSTEM

A number of principles can be derived from the preceding discussion of challenges and theories relevant to the development of an enabling system. Technical assistance and support services that comprise an enabling system for community development should:

Develop local control and competence. Decision making and planning should be localized to increase ownership of community problems and solutions. Local governments and, even more so, local voluntary associations need to be involved in the process. The skills and general capacity to follow through on the planning process are additional primary goals of the enabling system. This may include leadership training and providing opportunities for local groups to plan and decide.

Be flexible in the content areas. Enabling systems should support the changing and differing priorities and problems of the communities and organizations they serve. This does not require the enabling system to contain expertise in every possible issue. The enabling organization is aware of its own content strengths and it brokers clients to other systems where the content resources are available. The provision of information and referral services for organizational needs are essential. Training and assistance programs need to be developed based on community or organizational needs and requests rather than solely agency mandates.

Be provided as a sustained effort. Training and technical assistance interventions must be of significant duration and intensity to impact complex processes. "Low-dose" interventions such as one-shot generic workshops seldom produce sustained results. Workshops that follow participants through the program development and implementation process over several months or a year are more effective, especially if assistance is available between sessions.

Be experiential and practice/skills oriented. Concepts from adult education must be used to equip people with workable skills that are easily taught and readily usable. People learn best when they actually work on the problem. Simulations and field laboratories are effective methods.

Be problem-solving and results-oriented. Approaches should lead to tangible action plans based on a realistic assessment of both current and desired conditions of client organizations. Educational and skill-building programs must address actual problems experienced by participants. Learning will occur through actual experience addressing the problem.

Account for developmental phases of an organization. Different processes and issues are salient for mobilization, maintenance and mission phases of an organization. Educational programs and other forms of assistance should focus on the developmental phase of the organization. For example, community organizing training should be broken up over time to reflect the specific stage of the organizing experienced by participants (e.g., recruiting members, community assessment, planning, etc.).

Promote self-assessment of strengths and weaknesses. Services should efficiently address needs while not redundantly training for existing strengths. Client organizations must develop the capacity to identify and solve problems on their own with minimal outside support. Self-administered check list on necessary organization components (by-laws, newsletter, agendas, subcommittees) is an example.

Be adaptable to different "dose strengths." Services are gauged to the organization's needs and resource-center capacity (e.g., three pages of printed materials on meeting management or a half-day workshop as needed).

Be readily available and "on-line." Implementation is facilitated and learning leveraged by responding in a timely fashion to emergent needs. Toll-free numbers, "hot" lines, electronic bulletin boards, and regular evening office hours are some of the ways to make support services more accessible.

Promote resource sharing and networking among similar organizations. Resource exchange networks are among the most effective mechanisms for supporting voluntary organizations (Sarason & Lorentz, 1979).

Have active monitoring and outreach. Regular monitoring by phone or in person should be planned. Publicity, recognition and incentives for achievements should be embedded in the system.

Be sensitive to conflicts internal to local communities and sponsoring organizations. This should be a target for preventative action in enabling system planning and operations. Consultation skills must be developed. The distribution of awards, travel and other benefits of the technical assistance relationship must be carefully scrutinized. Whenever possible, collective efforts and groups rather than individuals should be awarded.

Facilitate information flow and feedback. The enabling system can develop mechanisms and techniques to assist community organizations in efficiently receiving information on their environment. Different types of mechanisms can be made available, including: assistance in the planning, implementation, and interpretation of needs and strengths assessments; evaluation assistance; resources for planning and evaluation; a monitoring system that can be accessed by community groups; and process evaluations with a feedback component as described in Chavis and Florin (1990).

Foster the use of local resources. Often groups served by national and regional organizations focus outside their community for resources and ideas and become overly dependent on technical assistance providers. This includes the dissemination of technical assistance and training skills and resources to local community staff and leadership.

Encourage innovation and adaptation. The development of new models, strategies and solutions must be endemic to the system so that programs can adapt to changes in their communities and be able to meet new challenges. Client organizations should be viewed as incubators of creative solutions. The diffusion of innovations will be enhanced by the creation of environments that are supportive of change and sustained through linkages within the network and among other networks or systems.

Provide resources for purposes of maintenance and production. The system should provide resources equally for (a) organizational development and maintenance (e.g., general assistance in community mobilization and coalition development, leadership development, organizational capacity building, etc.) and (b) for the production of activities that will achieve organizational goals (e.g., dissemination of effective health promotion strategies, programs, and curriculum). One organization does not need to develop expertise in all maintenance and production areas; expertise and responsibility, however, should be contained within the system and all members need to be aware of available resources. The system needs to build incentives and easily useable resources for purposes of maintenance.

SUPPORT FOR ENABLING SYSTEMS

There is a wide range of federal, state, and private foundation programs that incorporate many of the strategies described in this article. This is especially true in regards to efforts to collaborative, multisectoral initiatives that address substance abuse. The federal government has allocated $44 million dollars to the "Community Partnership Demonstration Program" to support programs in 150 communities, the Robert Wood Johnson Foundation has committed

$27 million to 15 communities as part of their "Fighting Back" program. There a variety of state and local efforts to engage all sectors of a community to respond to their substance abuse programs.

The Henry J. Kaiser Family Foundation had recruited an array of national partners to launch community health promotion programs and a corresponding enabling system in seven southern states and the District of Columbia. The Ford Foundation, the Charles Stewart Mott Foundation, and community foundations across the country are developing support systems for neighborhood organizations in low income communities to address social and economic issues. In Memphis, TN, the Free the Children Program and in Camden, NJ, the Alliance for the 21st Century are examples of enabling systems that are being developed to address the chronic poverty within neighborhoods using comprehensive and multi-level approaches. There is an impressive amount of momentum behind these approaches.

CHALLENGES FOR HUMAN SERVICES EDUCATION

The main challenge for human service education is training professionals to staff these systems, developing the technologies for these enabling systems and organizations, and developing an enabling system infrastructure that can endure beyond a current "fad."

There is a need to train and re-train human service and community development professionals for roles in these support systems. Experienced community organizers, community development consultants, and technical assistance providers need to reconsider their current strategies so that they can serve numerous communities and develop the appropriate skills as outlined in this article. We need to develop professionals who can "train trainers of trainers" in methods consistent with methods of adult education. These skills should not be taken for granted or assumed that good intentions and a flip chart will develop them. Professional schools of Social Work, Public Health and Urban Planning should provide skill building courses in adult education, group facilitation, information and referral methods, consultation skills and others.

There is a tremendous need to develop professionals with skills to support community initiatives in the areas of health promotion, community development, prevention, community mental health, family support systems, child care and many other areas. The most critical challenge in the area of training is the recruitment of students who see this area as a viable career opportunity. With the diminishing number of community organization programs, a new approach is needed that reflects the current and expected strategies in the area that was once considered community organization. This article demonstrates one significant strategy area that has evolved from earlier approaches. The approach presented in this article reflects a combination of the social action, social planning and locality development approaches outlined by Rothman (1968). The enabling system integrates all three approaches and therefore requires a professional with more integrated systems intervention skills as described in this article.

Many of these skills (e.g., adult education, grant management and resource development, technology, development and technology transfer,) may require the use of resources and experts outside of traditional social service disciplines. Such fields as cooperative extension, information science, business administration and education often have the personnel that can assist in training students and provide continuing education opportunities for current professionals. Most of the persons who will be employed in these systems will be experienced professionals and continuing education opportunities must be provided.

CONCLUSIONS

There is a multitude of opportunities to engage citizens through their communities in a collective problem solving process. The article presented a framework to organize a support system for these numerous community initiatives called an enabling system. This approach organizes theory, research, and the emerging experience of the authors and many other supportive organizations in a manner that can serve as a blueprint for the design of such a system. The framework presented offers an holistic approach to the development and maintenance of community mobilization. This article was not presented as a definitive statement, but rather as a starting point for research and practice. There is a need for widespread experimentation as well as documentation of existing efforts.

This approach provides a challenge to social welfare administrators and policy makers. The implementation of this approach will necessitate staff training, collaboration with other agencies, and a genuine partnership with grassroots community leaders. The strategy presented provides a vitally needed role for formal service delivery systems to support community organization and to add momentum to the tides of change.

REFERENCES

Argyris, C. Putnam, R., Smith, D.M. *Action science.* San Francisco: Jossey-Bass Publishers, 1985.

Bandura, A. *Social foundations of thought and action*: A social cognitive theory. Englewood Cliffs, NJ: Prentice Hall, 1986.

Bernstein, A.. A comparison of systematic and personal characteristics that support self-help groups. *American Journal of Community Psychology* (in press).

Bernstein, K. & Yin, R.K. *Evaluation of the Fund for Neighborhood Initiatives: Second year report.* Washington, DC: COSMOS Corporation, 1987.

Berrien, S.K. *General and social systems.* New Brunswick, NJ: Rutgers University Press, 1968.

Braithwaite, R.L., Murphy, F., Lythcott, N. & Blumenthal, D.S. Community organization and development for health promotion within an urban black community: A conceptual model. *Health and Education*, 1989, *20*, 56-60.

Chavis, D.M. *Report on the feasibility of a community development support system.* New Brunswick, NJ: Center for Community Education, 1990.

Chavis, D.M. & Florin, P. *Sustaining voluntary community organizations through action research.* Unpublished manuscript. New Brunswick, NJ: Center for Community Education, 1990.

Christenson, J.A. & Robinson, J.W. *Community Development in America.* Ames, IA: The Iowa State University Press, 1980.

Cook, S. Network structures from an exchange perspective. In P.V. Marsden & N. Lin (Eds.) *Social structure and network analysis.* Beverly Hills: Sage, 1982.

Curtis, L. (Ed.) (1987) Policies to prevent crime: Neighborhood, family, and employment strategies. *Annals of the American Academy of Political and Social Science, 494:* pp. 9-53.

Fawcett, S.B. et al. Creating and using social technologies for community empowerment. *Journal of Prevention in the Human Services*, 1984, *3*, 145-171.

Fischer, C.S. et al. *Networks and places.* New York: Free Press, 1977.

Florin, P. et al. A systems approach understanding and enhancing grassroots organizations: The block booster project. In R. Levine & Fitzgerald (Eds.), *Analysis of dynamic psychological systems.* New York: Plenum (in press).

Florin, P., Chavis, D.M. *Factors contributing to maintenance in block associations: A systemic view.* Unpublished manuscript, University of Rhode Island, 1990.

Florin, P. (1989) *Nurturing the grassroots: Neighborhood volunteer organizations and America's cities.* New York: Citizens Committee for New York City, 1989.

Freire, P. *The politics of education.* S. Hadley, MA: Bergin and Garvey, 1985.

Freire, P. *Pedagogy of the oppressed.* New York: Herder and Herder, 1970.

Gamm, L. & Fisher, F. (1980) The technical assistance approach. In J.A. Christenson & J.W. Robinson, Jr. (Eds.), *Community development in America.* Ames, IA: Iowa State University Press, 1980.

Garkovich, L.E. (1989) Local organizations and leadership in community development. In J.A. Christenson and J.W. Robinson (Eds) *Community development in America.* Ames, IA: Iowa State University Press. 196-218.

Gouldner, A.W. The norm of reciprocity: A preliminary statement. *American Sociological Review*, 1960, *25*, 161-179.

Granovetter, M. The strength of weak ties: A network theory revisited. In P.V. Marsden & N. Lin (Eds.), *Social structure and network analysis.* Beverly Hills: Sage, 1982.

Granovetter, M. The strength of weak ties. *American Journal of Sociology*, 1973, *78*, 1360-1380.

Green, L.W. The theory of participation: A qualitative analysis of its expression in national and international health policies. *The Advances in Health Education and Promotion*, 1986, *1*, 211-236.

Julien, T.M. *The relationship between self-help groups and the community organizations that provide their resources.* Unpublished doctoral dissertation, Columbia University, 1988.

Katz, D. & Kahn, R.L. *The social psychology of organizations* (2nd ed.). New York: Wiley, 1978.

Knowles, M.S. *The adult learner: A neglected species* (2nd ed.). Houston: Gulf Publishing Co., 1978.

Knowles, M.S. *The modern practice of adult education.* New York: City Press, 1970.

Knox, A.B. *Helping adults learn.* San Francisco: Jossey-Bass, 1986.

Levi-Strauss, C. *Elementary structures of kinship.* Boston: Beacon Press, 1969.

Lin, N. Social resources and instrumental action. In P.V. Marsden & N. Lin (Eds.), *Social structure and network analysis.* Beverly Hills: Sage, 1982.

Madera, E.J. A comprehensive systems approach to promoting mutual AIDS self-help groups: The New Jersey self-help clearing house model. *Journal Voluntary Action Research*, 1986, *15*, 57-63.

Marsden, P.V. & Lin, N. (Eds.) *Social structure and network analysis.* Beverly Hills: Sage, 1982.

Marsden, P.V. Brokerage behavior in restricted exchange networks. In P.V. Marsden & N. Lin (Eds.), *Social structure and network analysis.* Beverly Hills: Sage, 1982.

Maton, K.I. et al. Factors affecting the birth and death of mutual help groups: The role of national affiliation, professional involvement, and member focal problem. *American Journal of Community Psychology*, 1989, *17*, 643-671.

Merino, R.P. Fischer, E.P. & Bosch, S. (1985) Technical assistance offered to community health programs through a resource model. *Public Report*, 1985, *100*, 30.

Moynihan, D.P. *Family and Nation.* San Diego: Harcourt Brace Jovanovich, 1986.

Moynihan, D.P. *Maximum feasible misunderstanding.* New York: Free Press, 1969.

Murrell, S. (1973). *Community Psychology and social systems.* New York: Behavioral Publications.

Naparstek, A.J., Beigel, D.E. & Spiro, H.R. (1982) *Neighborhood networks for humane mental health care.* New York: Plenum.

Parcel, G.S., Taylor, W.C., Brink, S.G., Gottlieb, N., Engquist, K., O'Harra, N.M. & Erikson, M.F. 1989. Translating theory into practice: Intervention strategies for the diffusion for the health promotion innovation. *Family and community health, 12* (1) (3), 1-13.

Plas, J.P.M. *Systems psychology in the schools.* New York: Pergamon Press, 1986.

Prestby, J. & Wandersman, A. An empirical exploration of a framework of organizational viability: Maintaining block organizations. *Journal of Applied Behavioral Sciences*, 1985, *21*, 287-305.

Rich, R.C. Municipal services and the interaction of the voluntary and governmental sectors. *Administration and Society*, 1981, *13*, 59-76.

Rich, R.C. The roles of neighborhood organizations in urban service delivery. *Urban Affairs Papers*, 1979, *1*, 81-93.

Robinson, E.R. *Guide to networking.* New Brunswick, NJ: Center for Community Education, 1986.

Rogers, B.E. *Diffusion innovations* (3rd ed.). New York: Free Press, 1983.

Rothman, J. *Using research in organizations.* Beverly Hills: Sage, 1980.

Rothman, J. (1968) Three models of community organization practice, *Social work practice 1968* Columbia University Press, 16-47.

Sanders, I. The social reconnaissance method of community study. *Research in Rural Sociology and Development*, 1985, *2*, 235-255.

Sarason, S.P.B. et al. *Human services and resource networks.* San Francisco: Jossey-Bass, 1977.

Sarason, S.P.B. & Lorentz, E. *The challenge of the resource network*. San Francisco: Jossey-Bass, 1979.

Spiegel, H. Coproduction in the context of neighborhood development, *Journal of Voluntary Action Research*, 1987, *16*.

Varela, J.P. *Introduction to social science technology*. New York: Academic Press, 1970.

Vidal, A.P.C., Howitt, A.M., & Foster, K.P. (1986) *Stimulating community report: An assessment of the local initiative support corporation*. Cambridge, MA: John F. Kennedy School of Government, 1986.

Von Bertalanffy, L. An outline of general system theory. *British Journal of Social Science*, 1950, *1*, 34-65.

Washnis, G.J. *Community development strategies: Case studies of major model cities*. New York: Praeger, 1974.

Wellman, B. Studying personal communities. In P.V. Marsden, & N. Lin (Eds.), *Social structure network analysis*. Beverly Hills: Sage, 1982.

Yates, D. *Neighborhood democracy*. Lexington, MA.: D.C. Heath, 1973.

Building High Access
Community Organizations:
Structures As Strategy

Jacqueline B. Mondros, DSW
Scott M. Wilson, PhD

Most analysts of community organizing agree that the major re-source of social action organizations (Grosser & Mondros, 1984) as they exert pressure for social change is a large base of committed activists which both legitimize and empower the organization to act (Haggstrom, 1987). Problems organizers have in attaining and then maintaining people's involvement are illustrated by Burghardt (1984):

> An organizer offers a familiar complaint: one million people show up in New York in June, 1984 for an anti-nuclear rally. It is the largest march in U.S. history, writes the activist; but three months later organizing activity is at a snail's pace. (p. 31)

The work organizers do to involve people is what Brager and Specht (1973) and others (Fisher, 1984) refer to as "building the base." Involving, engaging, and sustaining a large and strongly

Dr. Mondros is Associate Dean, Barry University School of Social Work, 11300 N.E. Second Ave., Miami Shores, FL 33161. Dr. Wilson is Educational Specialist, Council on Social Work Education, 1600 Duke Street, Suite 300, Alexandria, VA 22314.

An earlier version of this paper was presented at the Association on Community Organization and Social Administration Symposium, Annual Program Meeting, Council on Social Work Education, Chicago, 1989.

identified group of participants is important to achieving organizational goals.

In this article, we describe problems organizers typically face in engaging and maintaining people, and suggest why such difficulties have persisted. We propose that organizers use their organizational structures consciously to mitigate some of these problems. We present ideas for promoting access and offer examples of current organizing efforts consistent with them.

METHODOLOGY

This article is based on a descriptive study of 42 social action organizations located along the Eastern seaboard. These organizations spanned the urban to rural continuum; operated at local, city, metropolitan, state, and national levels; were comprised of people with a variety of ethnic and social class experiences; and worked on many different social issues and agendas. The organizations were identified reputationally. To meet study criteria, the organizations had to have a membership, be at least two years old and have at least one full-time staff member who had been employed by the organization for at least one year. We required that the organizations' primary purpose be to pressure for change, and they had to be actively organizing around one or more issues. The lead organizers, of which ten were MSW social workers, completed a questionnaire on organizational variables, and took part in a partially structured interview focused on the organizing process. A key volunteer participant took part in a similar interview, providing a member perspective. Given the purposive sample and limited number of organizations included, findings and conclusions are not generalized beyond the groups studied. Data are examined in greater depth in a forthcoming text (Mondros & Wilson).

PROBLEMS WITH PARTICIPATION

Recruiting, engaging, and maintaining participants receives a great deal of attention in many organizing texts (Brager & Specht, 1979; Henderson & Thomas, 1980; Twelvetrees, 1982; Staples, 1984). In our interviews with them, an overwhelming number of organizers also thought these were critical areas, and commonly complained about several difficulties they faced in recruiting, engaging, and maintaining participants.

One frequent comment was about how difficult it is to find people who are interested in the issues of progressive social action organizations. Organizers bemoan that even among those who are interested, few people are prepared to work actively for change. Organizers also complain that too often they are unable to attract the "right kind" of people to their organizations, particularly those who would bring valuable talents or traits. Often, this theme is expressed by organizers who find themselves unable to recruit people of color who could bolster the organization's claim of representativeness.

There are also worries about the prospects of engaging people in the organization and its work. Many organizers complain that people are either unwilling to assume roles or could not perform them adequately because they lack skills or live far from the organization's headquarters. Other organizers worry that some people accept organizational roles as a way of maintaining their power and control, then resist including others in organizational decision making and planning. Consequently, newcomers are excluded from taking on responsibility. Organizers commonly bemoan the time they spend negotiating internal conflicts, managing member relationships, or finding and training someone to take on organizational responsibilities.

Finally, organizers mourn those people who are interested, agree to take on roles, but then disappear. Sometimes people join because of self-interest in an issue and leave after their problem is solved, never embracing more collective and on-going interests in a way that makes them most valuable to the organization. Other people "burn out" after a period of activism, either because they are frustrated with a lack of progress or because other life events take precedence. Organizers bemoan the resulting difficulties in building on-going campaigns with people who are often "missing in action," as well as the passivity of participants who continue as members but do not deepen and extend their investment by taking initiative or leadership roles.

Often organizers' complaints reflect very real environmental obstacles to participation. It has always been difficult for people to travel to take part in national, regional, and state-wide activities at remote headquarters. But even local organizers have seen a change in the participation patterns of their members (Mondros & McGuffin, in press). Changes in the economy, particularly the need to work or to work more, have already made people less available for community participation. One organizer told us, "It used to be that at least some people were home during the day—women, senior citizens, people working nights or swing shift. We can't do things during the day now, and it's harder to get them out for evening meetings. Everyone has to work."

Organizing requires a large group of activists, but economic and social realities restrict the ability of many people to even begin to participate in social action organizations. When people do participate, they invariably and appropriately bring their own agendas, questions, and status needs which create additional demands on the organizer. Some organizers experience these member demands as interfering in their work. Like librarians who grudgingly accept those who borrow "their" books, some organizers are frustrated by the people who comprise "their" organizations. They do not learn to accommodate to their members' demands and, therefore, question how much time and energy should be expended on recruiting and working with participants.

We argue that many organizers hold biases which predispose them to be inattentive to members (Mondros & Wilson, 1990). First, many organizers articulate goals for substantive change, not member development, suggesting their priorities are for outcomes, not involvement. For these organizers, working with members is viewed as a diversion from issue and strategy work, only indirectly related to the substantive gains on issues they seek. Second, some organizers appear to believe that true commitment cannot be developed, and that people who have to be convinced are, by definition, less reliable members. Thus, these organizers only pay attention to those already converted, doing little recruitment or member development work. Third, organizers have an acute sense of the importance of their own expertise to the organization. Their status is primarily a reflection of their expert knowledge. Consequently, these organizers may see recruiting and working with unskilled participants as potentially presumptuous threats to their own power in the organization. The competing time demands organizers face on the job may also dissuade them from doing recruitment and member development work. Working with members takes time and effort, requires interactive skills rather than issue expertise, is never-ending and often frustrating, and requires organizers to have continual contact with strangers who may disagree with them.

Each of these reasons predispose organizers to issue work, with minimal attention to involving people. Organizers may not realize that they are signaling that the organization can function effectively without participants, that it is in the capable hands of the staff, confirming people's notions that non-involvement, passivity, and episodic engagement are acceptable.

As noted previously, the current socio-economic context makes it inherently difficult for organizers to find and maintain members. This difficulty is exacerbated when organizers themselves are ambivalent or neglectful about giving attention to member participation. Some organizers complain of lack of participation, but are bewildered about what might change this. Others, however, readily acknowledge these difficulties and consciously try to ameliorate them. Expanding on the ideas of these latter organizers, when organizers view structure strategically and consciously use it to recruit, engage, and maintain an active group of people they can mitigate some of the inherent restraints against participation.

ORGANIZATIONAL STRUCTURE AND INVOLVEMENT

Brager and Holloway (1978) define structure as "the ways in which the members of an organization are arranged in relation to one another, the prescribed relationships and rules, either formal or informal, that define organizational authority and responsibility" (p. 20). Social action organizations, like others, have rules, roles, division of labor, and patterns of communication. Social action organizations also may have distinctive features. To the extent that these organizations may be more non-hierarchical than others, authority may be democratically vested in the membership, and there may be mutual accountability among staff and members. These features serve to underscore the sense of ownership and stake members have in the organization. The question is how organizers can best define and use organizational structures so that people want to participate, increasingly feel a sense of stake in the group, and continue their involvement.

The conscious use of structure to further goal attainment is discussed in the organizational theory literature. Ullrich and Wieland (1980) use the term "structural responsiveness" to refer to the ability to purposively design and implement new organizational structures. Organizational theorists stressed controlling behavior with structure (Katz & Kahn, 1960). Human relationists and organizational humanists promoted using structure to enhance positive participation (Roethlisberger & Dickson, 1949; McGregor, 1960; Likert, 1967), including such concepts as "psychological contracting" which bind people to organizational goals (Dunahee & Wrangler, 1974), extrinsic and intrinsic rewards for members (Reif, 1975), and open and interactive systems (Lawrence & Lorsch, 1967). Although conscious use of structure is not often discussed in the organizing literature (Brager & Specht, 1973), these ideas from organizational theory provide the conceptual impetus for organizers to create structures which build and maintain participation.

HIGH ACCESS ORGANIZATIONS

The relationship between members and social action organizations is interactional. Because social action organizations are voluntary associations, ultimately members define the length and depth of their relationship with the organization. When they are dissatisfied, they drop out or disrupt activities. Yet, it is also true that by using organizational structures which encourage participation, social action organizers have shown that they can positively influence individuals' interactions by either encouraging or dissuading participation.

If social action organizations are to involve people, access to the organization and its leadership structure become the primary concern. Recognizing that there are real environmental obstacles to participation, organizers need to craft organizations which are as inviting, open, and "user friendly" as possible. Such organizations promote "high access" because they are consciously designed to make it easy for people to join, to find personal and social "niches" within the organization, to take on responsibility and maintain their allegiance, and to progress to higher levels of responsibility and leadership. Consequently, they counter the problems social action organizations typically have in involving and maintaining people.

In our view, social action organizations have structures which either enhance or minimize participation. Structures that involve people, which facilitate initial joining and subsequent involvement, we call *bridges*. They enable recruits to make the transition from "outsider" to organizational insider, and from member to leader. Structures which impede involvement or entree to leadership positions we call *barriers*, and those which move people to new statuses or positions in the organization we call *gates*. Gates allow some people to move into the leadership group by meeting some predetermined criteria, while excluding others.

Staff and existing leadership in high access organizations consciously design and maintain bridges which seek to bring new members into the organization, and increasingly involve them in its leadership structure. Some examples of bridge-building techniques are: calculated and thorough outreach and recruitment; the existence of orientations, mentoring or buddy systems which link new people to organizational ventures and veterans; the availability of participatory and decision-making roles; meetings which are held at accessible times and places; and methods of soliciting member ideas and interests.

At the same time, high access organizations assiduously avoid such obvious barriers to involvement as formal restrictions for membership or voting, inflexible criteria or processes for selecting people for leadership positions, and inaccessible meeting times and places. They also steer clear of the more subtle barriers such as haphazard or non-existent recruitment, use of insiders' jargon, reliance on traditional or long-standing leadership, narrowly controlled decisions, and one-way and limited communications.

Finally, high access organizations construct gates for two reasons. First, they are used sparingly to ensure that the most important organizational roles (e.g., chairperson or treasurer) are filled by the most able people. More often, gates are used to facilitate the passage of new members from minimal levels of involvement to more intensive and complex roles and responsibilities. Examples of organizational gates are the use of training programs or proven accomplishments as criteria for assuming leadership positions.

We offer some ideas and examples of how barriers to participation have been avoided and bridges and gates established to recruit new people, engage them initially, maintain them, and develop them as members and leaders.

RECRUITMENT

Few social action organizations have strict eligibility requirements which exclude people intentionally. Yet such inclusiveness does not mean the organization is accessible to all people who could join. There are commonly more subtle barriers to involvement. It is often difficult for people, including those who may be sympathetic to the issues, to locate — let alone affiliate with — an organization working on their concerns. Leaflets and posters need to be seen to be acted on, and they have to offer meaning to the reader. Even if people attend an organizational event such as a demonstration, they probably will not learn about on-going possibilities for participation, nor be told how to contact the organization which has sponsored the event. Nor can organizers always ask all the people attending these events for their names and phone numbers so they can be re-contacted.

Organizers can consciously counteract these recruitment barriers and build bridges in several ways.

1. *Calculate who is likely to participate and target recruitment accordingly.* The people who are most likely to become active in an organization are not always the nearest, most accessible, nor most obvious ones. Periodically, organizers can re-think who might be interested in participating and why. Opinion polls, formal surveys of members or drop-outs, and conversations with community leaders are ways of defining such a pool, and efforts then can be made to engage their participation. This targeted recruitment may generate as many members as the time honored method of distributing leaflets on street corners or the costly approach of purchasing mailing lists.

A recent example of such calculated recruitment was evident in the summer of 1989, as the Pennsylvania legislature was again debating the State's abortion law. Opinion polls consistently show that the strongest pro-abortion sentiment was among Jewish women. For the first time pro-choice organizers consciously and specifically recruited from synagogue sisterhoods in the major cities. Busloads of these women attended demonstrations at the State Capitol, noticeably swelling the ranks of the protesters. Most of them had never been active before. No one, it seems, had ever asked them, nor developed a bridge which encouraged their participation.

2. *Create and communicate messages* designed specifically for potential participant pools. Different audiences require different appeals which respond to their unique interests, concerns, and reservations. Instead of a single message for all people and all occasions (e.g., "a standard rap") organizers will have to tune into each audience and craft a message which builds a bridge directly to their experience. For example, when recruiting a neighborhood businessman an organizer will stress the commercial advantages of his increased visibility in the community, while an appeal to low income residents would focus on their immediate needs for better housing.

3. *Use multiple recruitment methods* to attract and build bridges to the greatest possible number of recruits. Face-to-face recruitment by friends and family are the most effective way of generating new people, but presentations to other groups or as a part of service provision are also valuable. Flyers and posters are best used to locate and connect with people who are not part of identified networks.

The Parish Ministry or congregational organizing approach (Boyte, 1990) is a model which combines calculated recruitment, specifically designed messages, and multiple recruitment methods. The membership pool of these organizations is defined as the community's churches and synagogues which become the member groups of the organization. In this way the organization is built on large numbers of people who come as members of a group with shared beliefs and concerns. The organizations use religious teachings and liturgy to support social justice issues and underscore the need for community organizing. Recruitment messages stress that members define themselves and behave as "communities of faith."

People are recruited first by the pastor or rabbi (through conversations with the clergy, announcements from the pulpit), and later by other members of the congregation. Religiously unaffiliated people are reached through presentations to other groups such as civic associations and senior citizen groups, press coverage about the organization, and flyers distributed to homes and schools. The bridges to the organization are readily available to members of local churches and synagogues, and still not denied other community members.

4. *Recognize recruitment deficits.* Despite their best efforts, organizers may not be able to attract everyone, not even those to whom they most want to appeal. According to many organizers it is especially difficult to build bridges to poor and minority constituencies with issues such as feminism and environmental causes. Even all the techniques mentioned previously will have only modest success, and some entirely new approach may be needed.

One innovative approach is exemplified by a relationship formed between a state-wide environmental action organization and a local community group in Harlem. An environmental group located in rural New York, addresses a broad array of environmental issues. It is successful in recruiting members through political activities, celebrations, and Hudson River cruises. Although it defines its constituency as all the people living along the Hudson River, the organization has basically a white middle class membership, and has consistently failed to attract poor and minority participants. At the same time, an African-American organization in Harlem was organizing against the building of a sewage plant on its waterfront. The environmental group began a consulting relationship with the Harlem group, advising them on several campaigns. In this way environmental activism is extended into an area and with a group which is not easily reached while both groups maintain their own identities and issues.

ENGAGEMENT

Newcomers will often take away an initial impression of their contact with an organization which will either deter or enhance their desire to return. They "size up" the other people present, determining whether or not this is a group with whom they will feel comfortable. Issues of race and class, as suggested above, are among the more obvious factors here. It is reassuring that someone known and trusted is there, and disconcerting if others in attendance are not introduced. Entering a new situation where everyone else seems to be "in the know" is alienating. History which is not recounted, complex information which is not explained, decisions which are made without rationales being offered, opinions which are not solicited, and roles which are not offered all serve to deter the involvement of newcomers, to create barriers rather than bridges.

With these barriers in mind, bridges can be consciously constructed to engage new participants in organizational work and connect them to other people:

1. *Repeated personal contacts* enhance the development of relationships between the recruit, current organizational members, and the organizer. These relationships ease the newcomer's transition into the organization. The newcomer is helped to get "on board" formally with both the organization's work and membership through briefings by the organizer or when assigned a veteran member as a mentor or buddy. Informally, opportunities for socializing and celebrations (e.g., holiday or victory parties) cement a sense of camaraderie and common stake in the organization. Through such repeated contacts, bridges are built to other participants, to a shared vision, and to the group as a whole.

2. *Orientation and training for new participants* can provide background information and skill training which allow new participants to feel capable of making contributions. Further, this approach is far more engaging and personal than merely distributing information packets. These programs bring new recruits into the current work of the organization, without forcing the established members to backtrack as well. Such introductions also suggest that newcomers are valued and expected to participate meaningfully in the organization.

3. *Easy access to committees with real work and decision-making authority* gives the message that the organization is truly owned and operated by members. The initial enthusiasm newcomers bring can be easily dampened when they are excluded from active involvement. When even the newest recruits are asked their opinions, work

alongside veteran members, and encouraged to take on responsibilities, the organization's interest and trust in their competence is expressed. Correspondingly, newcomers see they can immediately contribute. Established leaders should be given the responsibility for incorporating newcomers, to avoid being bored by repetition or threatened by the attention focused on newcomers.

Access problems have been especially troublesome for national organizations who must somehow engage people who may live a great distance away. To correct for this deficit, two organizations have developed "circuit rider" approaches where organizers travel to local groups, rather than expect members to come to central headquarters. In one case, a national organizer of a group which advocates on Latin American issues spends a short period of time working with a local chapter around an issue which has been defined nationally. When the mission is accomplished, the organizer may go on to another city or return to the national office. In this model, it is the organizer who bridges physical and interpersonal distance by bringing distant issues to people in local communities. In the second case, a national voting rights organization, solicits the participation or accepts invitations of local grassroots groups working on referendums, election reform, or some other issue which has electoral or legislative features. The organization sends an organizer to work intensively with the members of that local group to design, plan, and execute a registration campaign. The direction of the campaign, its goals, strategies, and targets, are always decided by people at the local level. The organizer maintains contact with the staff and leadership of these local organizations, and during national elections, helps them to coordinate their local register efforts. In this model, access is increased locally, bridges are built around local issues, but the national organization's goals are also achieved. Again, the organizer as circuit rider is the "glue" which holds the local efforts together.

MAINTAINING PARTICIPANTS

For people who have been successfully recruited and engaged, questions about continued involvement and opportunities for organizational leadership arise. If their assignments and responsibilities are not reflective of their interests and talents, they feel underutilized. If they are performing only menial chores, well below their level of desire and competence, they may even feel exploited and demeaned. If they receive no recognition or credit for their work, they feel ignored and unappreciated. With little sense of their role in and meaning to the organization, people simply drop out.

A long time board member of a city-wide tenants rights organization says,

> A few years ago I decided I wanted to get more familiar with the organization, so I figured I'd come in and answer telephones. . . . The telephone was answered before I could answer it. I quit because I didn't like it . . . I could do a lot of work if they would let me.

This woman's complaint is ironic given that organizers argue that for social action organizations to be successful people must be maintained in the organization and must increasingly accept greater responsibility. In fact, some organizers do little to maintain and increase the responsibility of participants, while others work to sustain only a "core" or "cadre" as organizational leaders. These organizers, believing they need only a few select people, do little to keep people motivated. They establish very rigid criteria and processes for moving into leadership, making it virtually impossible for anyone to assume a leader role. In these instances, there are few sustaining bridges and gates are used as barriers.

Instead, the bridges that have been built earlier between the organization and newcomers must be maintained and enhanced to encourage participants to tackle new tasks and challenges. It is also appropriate and realistic to establish some gates for the most important positions in the organization. It is foolhardy, for example, to have a chronic procrastinator as the organization's treasurer. On the other hand, the most articulate member does not always have to speak for the group; others can learn to do public speaking. Therefore, structural gates are functional for selecting people for the most crucial roles, and at the same time allowing access to most leader roles for as many people as possible. With this in mind, bridges and gates to sustain and deepen involvement can be developed:

1. *Offer opportunities for leadership to as many people as possible.* The organization should offer many opportunities for people to lead beyond the formal officer positions, and many people should be entitled to these roles. Positions on committees and task forces, assignments to do research or raise funds or recruit, and opportunities to do public speaking or public relations can be distributed to keep people engaged and active. People are given the sense that their work fits with and links to others', and that if they so choose, they can advance in the organization (Alinsky, 1969; Tjerandsen, 1980; Kahn, 1982; Staples, 1984).

2. *Help people take on and execute new roles.* On-going supports which give people the capability and confidence to carry out the tasks and roles cited above are the primary bridges and gates which sustain people and help them move into leader roles. For most people, leadership skills are not innate. People often approach leadership with ambivalence: they both want and are frightened of performing visible roles. Modeling, role playing, briefing, and on-going training are important ways to help people acquire these skills (Biklen, 1983; Staples, 1984). People also should be invited to reflect on their experiences, share their concerns, ask questions, admit to insecurities. Again, this helps to reconfirm that their ideas and comments are valued.

3. *Create and maintain rules which ensure that new leadership must be generated.* Established leaders cannot become entrenched in the top organizational positions if these positions are to be made available to new people. The organization must have rules governing leadership succession which limit terms and numbers of office which can be held, create emeritus positions for established leaders to move into (e.g., honorary president or board member), and require members to step out of positions for a period of time before being elected again (Staples, 1984). Ironically, organizers themselves often discourage leadership by usurping roles which could easily be performed by members. Rules which limit staff powers (e.g., mandating who speaks for the organization, who signs agreements with external actors) will curtail organizers' tendencies to preempt roles which leaders could appropriately perform.

4. *Build a reward system.* Reward systems are common in our culture, in corporate and voluntary organizations. Yet, some orga-

nizers believe that commitment is its own just reward. The ability to attain a level of distinction among their peers, to be honored for one's contribution, is certainly an incentive for many people to continue their participation. Reward giving in social action organizations appears to be mostly informal because these organizations seldom have the resources to go beyond sending thank you notes and/or holding a celebration which honors a members' efforts. Still, rewards should be distributed consciously so that they enhance the sense of group achievement and give recognition equitably. A group in Northern New Jersey which uses a congregational organizing approach, honors leaders during church and synagogue services, thereby increasing the visibility of the honor and enhancing the member's sense of distinction.

More formal reward systems should be considered as well. A city-wide group, for instance, negotiated with the City to build low-income housing units in Boston, and as a reward for participation, eligible members had first choice for unit selection. In this way, their participation had a real pay-off.

IMPLICATIONS FOR EDUCATION AND PRACTICE

For organizers to build the active participatory organizations they need and desire, they will need to begin to consider recruitment, engagement, and maintenance of people as strategy. Such organizers will construct high access organizations, i.e., they actively build bridges to reach people, assiduously avoid barriers which impede involvement, and make judicious use of gates to open opportunities for leadership to as many people as possible.

We have cited examples of social action organizations which have made conscious use of structure to increase participation. We have also offered some ideas for improving organizational access which are applicable to many organizations. Of course, each organization will have its own specific set of access problems which require creative solutions. Our hope is that our work will invite others who write about organizing to examine the effect of structure on outcomes. Teachers of organizing should help students analyze this area. Finally, we encourage organizers to be conscious about the accessibility of their organizations, to experiment with and refine the ideas offered here, and to find new ways of enhancing participation.

REFERENCES

Alinsky, S. *Reveille for radicals*. New York: Vintage Books, 1969.

Biklen, D. *Community organizing: Theory and practice*. Englewood Cliffs, NJ: Prentice-Hall, Inc., 1983.

Boyte, H. *Commonwealth*. New York: The Free Press, 1990.

Brager, G. & Holloway, S. *Changing human service organizations: Politics and practice*. New York: The Free Press, 1978.

Brager, G. & Specht, H. *Community organizing*. New York: Columbia University Press, 1973.

Burghardt, S. (1984). The strategic crisis of grass roots organizing. *Against the Current*, 1984, *3*, 31.

Dunahee, M. & Wrangler, L. The psychological contract: A conceptual structure for management/employee relations. *Personnel Journal*, 1974, *53*, 518-526.

Fisher, R. *Let the people decide*. Boston: Twayne Publishers, 1984.

Grosser, C. & Mondros, J. Pluralism and participation: The political action approach. In R. Roberts and S. Taylor (Eds.), *Theories and applications of community social work*. New York: Columbia University Press, 1984.

Haggstrom, W. The tactics of organization building. In F.M. Cox, J.L. Erlich, J. Rothman & J.E. Tropman (Eds.), *Strategies of community organization*. Itasca, IL: F.E. Peacock, 1987.

Henderson, P. & Thomas, D. *Skills in neighborhood work*. London: George Allen & Unwin, 1980.

Kahn, S. *Organizing: A guide for grassroots leaders*. New York: McGraw Hill, 1982.

Katz, D. & Kahn, R. *The social psychology of organizations*. New York: John Wiley and Sons, 1960.

Lawrence, P. & Lorsch, J. *Organization and environment*. Homewood, IL: Richard D. Irwin, 1967.

Likert, R. *The human organization: Its management and value*. New York: McGraw-Hill, 1967.

McGregor, D. *The human side of enterprise*. New York: McGraw-Hill, 1960.

Mondros, J.B. & McGuffin, N. Yonkers: A tale of two cities. In C. LeCroix (Ed.), *Casebook for Social Workers*. New York: The Haworth Press (in press).

Mondros, J.B. & Wilson, S.M. *Staying alive: Career selection and sustenance of community organizers. Administration in Social Work*, 1990, *14*, 95-109.

Mondros, J.B. & Wilson, S.M. *Organizing for empowerment*. New York: Columbia University Press (in press).

Reif, W. Intrinsic versus extrinsic rewards: Resolving the controversy. *Human Resource Management*, 1975, *14*, 2-10.

Roethlisberger, F. & Dickson, W. *Management and the worker*. Cambridge, MA: Harvard University Press, 1949.

Staples, L. *Roots to power*. New York: Praeger Press, 1984.

Tjerandsen, C. *Education for citizenship: A foundation's experience*. Santa Cruz, CA: Emil Schwarzhaupt Foundation, 1980.

Twelvetrees, A. *Community work*. London: The Macmillan Press, 1982.

Ullrich, R. & Wieland, G. *Organization theory and design*. Homewood, IL: Richard D. Irwin, 1980.

PART 2: UNDERSTANDING COMMUNITY PLANNING AND HUMAN SERVICE ORGANIZATIONS

Patterns of Organizing for Community Human Service Planning: A Statewide Survey

Ray H. MacNair, PhD

INTRODUCTION

The field of community organization needs a more solid foundation of empirically based knowledge and theory. Recent efforts to identify a theoretical framework have been unsuccessful (Taylor & Roberts, 1985). Rothman's (1974) compilation of empirical findings in 1974 was a major step in the right direction, but that kind of

Dr. MacNair is Associate Professor, School of Social Work, The University of Georgia, Athens, GA 30602.

An earlier version of this paper was presented at the Association on Community Organization and Social Administration Symposium, Annual Program Meeting, Council on Social Work Education, Atlanta, 1988.

effort has been neglected over the last sixteen years. To build knowledge and theory will require empirically derived theory and theoretically based empirical research. Little empirically based theory can be found. Germain's discussion of ecological theory is useful, for example, but it is non-empirical and avoids giving attention to the organizational component in community organization (Taylor & Roberts, 1985).

The objective of this article is to provide an example of theoretically derived research on community planning. It presents the empirical findings of a study which is theoretically relevant. It serves four purposes:

1. to test a creative survey methodology which is not expensive, suggesting more expensive improvements;
2. to present empirical findings on patterns of organization among community human service planning bodies in scarce and not so scarce resource environments and associations of these variables with reported levels of effectiveness;
3. to suggest explanatory theories which can be used in the quest for more rigorous conceptual and theoretical formulations of community organization practice;
4. to discuss the development of a theoretical focus for practitioners and students of community organization, which will ultimately serve to guide them in their practice.

The "ecological" theory of community organization, first introduced by Leiter and Webb (1983), is based on the analogy of organisms surviving in a resource environment. The field of "human ecology" was first established by Hawley, a sociologist, in 1950. This field refers to the exchange of power and resources between units within a community, between communities, and between a community and its environment. Ecological theory focuses attention on the community as a context in which resources are negotiated and exchanged (Hawley, 1950). A diagnosis of a community organization, therefore, includes an assessment of the availability of resources to it, the rules which govern their availability, and the power which is required to leverage those rules (Long, 1972).

Specifically, the theory focuses on the resources required by a community organization to achieve its goals, the points of leverage over resources in the social environment which it proposes to pursue, and the strategies for pursuing the requisite resources.

BACKGROUND

A review of the literature reveals that cross-sectional quantitative studies of community human service planning groups have rarely been done. The literature is replete with prescriptive books and articles which offer models of organization for planning, ideal typical approaches to collective decision making, technical forms of scheduling, systematic techniques of data gathering for needs assessments, model strategies for citizen or client participation, and exemplary roles of social planners (Lauffer, 1978; Cox et al., 1977; Rubin, 1986; Brager, 1987; Lauffer, 1982). Case studies have been published which bring these models down to earth (Ecklein, 1983; Rothman et al., 1976), but little effort has been made to document across a range of communities what actually happens when natural cases are selected for observation, rather than exemplary models (Shostak, 1966; Kramer, 1967; Verma, 1986).

Roland Warren (1974) studied coordination, participation, and innovation in Model Cities communities in the early 1970s. A study by Callahan (1973) revealed obstacles to planning in nine metropolitan cities. MacNair (1983) analyzed a sample of citizen participation groups according to the terms of social exchange and power theory. He found low status, low power organizations more open to meaningful input from citizen participants, presumably because of their greater need to garner support for their programs.

Funding for such studies has not generally been available in recent years, but the difference between empirical fact and the ideal model is especially crucial in the early 1990s. Increasingly cynical local community participants need to be told honestly what can actually be accomplished by organizing and what kind of organizing works for a given set of purposes.

The prevailing conservatism in American politics, the federal decision-making apparatus, and deficit reduction requirements place increasing pressure on local communities to document human service problems and mobilize voluntary community wide support to meet needs minimally. It is vital that local procedures be established to document problems (Neuber, 1982) and that local people be involved in responding to the information. When predicted crises accumulate, as they are now, planning, development, and lobbying activities already in place will facilitate a constructive response.

THE SETTING

An immediate purpose of this quantitative study, administered in 1987, is to examine how the field of community human service planning is actually practiced in Georgia. Georgia's state agencies had not enacted a statewide local planning procedure which would serve to instigate the development of local organizations. In this sense, it is virgin territory. Any programs identified in this study arise from voluntary initiative alone.

Georgia is well known for its southern rural culture. Forty percent of its six million population, however, lives in one region, the Atlanta Metropolitan Area, which is rapidly urbanizing the entire northwestern sector of the state. On the other hand, the state has 159 counties, nearly two-thirds of which have fewer than 20,000 people.

Poverty is well distributed throughout the state. The smaller counties have higher *rates* of poverty, however. Two-thirds of the counties with less than 20,000 population have rates of poverty above twenty percent, according to the 1980 Census; less than one-third of the larger counties have that rate. The smaller counties have lower rates of per capita income. They have lower proportions of managerial personnel in the labor force, lower proportions of professional workers, and lower overall levels of education. In short, they have lesser pools of resources in wealth and human occupational talent than do the larger counties, after adjusting for size. The indicators of human suffering and need are higher in the smaller counties. The question is raised, therefore, how will resources be leveraged and developed to meet those needs when the available human resources and monetary resource pools are relatively small?

In this context, the more general question is, how do community planning organizations operate in order to make use of the resources that are available in their environment? Are there some resource planning patterns identifiable and is there a pattern or style of operation which appears to be more effective than others? To address these questions, the following methodology was developed.

METHODOLOGY

Community human service planning organizations in Georgia are not organized nor are they listed on any statewide listing. No state agency has initiated model community planning activities. This study is focused on natural, locally spontaneous (indigenous) groups and organizations. As a result, there is no one local official who can be contacted. A brief questionnaire was sent to each of five to eight formally identifiable officials in each of the 159 counties in Georgia: the welfare director, the mental health director, the school superintendent, the county clerk, the city clerk of the county seat, a hospital director, the director of the Chamber of Commerce, and the director of the United Way. This form provided a definition of "organizations for community resources planning in the human services" and asked for contact information on any such groups which were identifiable within the county. The definition included three elements: multi-organizational combinations, an exchange of information concerning human service needs, and an effort to establish policies or resources to meet those needs.

When at least three of these forms were returned from a county reporting that no such group existed, it was concluded that no planning group existed. Callbacks were made if no clear information came in, with limited success. Ultimately, 23 counties did not respond; they are listed as non-response counties. Fifty counties responded negatively, reporting that no planning group existed. Full second stage questionnaires were sent to 86 counties, 30 of which failed to return them with appropriate responses. They are also non-response counties. Fifty-six counties returned correct responses on the second stage forms. These 56 counties plus the 50 reporting affirmatively that they have no planning group yield a response rate of 67%. The 56 counties with planning organizations which responded fully are relatively urbanized counties compared with the non-response counties. The urban bias in this sample probably minimizes urban-rural differences.

The fifty-six fully responding counties reported 130 planning organizations and documented the characteristics and experience of one planning venture for each of the 130 organizations. Random illustrations of these groups and their ventures are given as follows:

In Tift County, a south central community of 37,000, a planning committee sponsored by United Way engaged a broad range of institutions in an effort to develop day care programs for the elderly. A Children's Interagency Council was organized in Thomas County, a deep south Georgia community of 44,000 that worked to develop educational programs on parenting for child abusers. Their interagency involvement was relatively narrow, however. Talbot, a west central rural community of less than seven thousand, has an Interagency Council which is broad based in its organizing pattern. They worked on mapping bus stops for a rural transportation system.

Screven County, a community of 15,000 in east central Georgia, has a narrowly organized management team which worked on developing clothing and food programs in emergency assistance. A metropolitan community of 203,000 in east central Georgia, centered in Richmond County, formed a broad based but informal network which met to advocate for youth and older worker job programs through JTPA. Dekalb County, in the Atlanta Metropolitan Area, has a population of roughly 440,000. The county government legislates the broad based formation of a human services planning commission. They reported participating in a voluntary council in Atlanta to map out shelter programs for the homeless in the Atlanta region.

These illustrations reveal an assortment of different kinds of goals in varying forms of organization. There is no strict difference between urban and rural areas, but general variations are certainly expected.

As a contextual measure, counties were classified as urban or rural based on size (20,000 and over vs. under 20,000), representing resource environments of the planning groups. The questionnaire data were used to formulate three types of measures, (1) initiating variables, (2) organizational practices, and (3) outcome.

Initiating Variables

Initiating variables are those that clearly precede and set the stage for the planning outcomes. They are the organizational *form* of a planning organization: bureaucratically *mandated* (governmental board, interagency management team, or staff team) or *voluntary* (council or network) and a planning *goal: direct service* or *procedural change*. Examples of procedural change goals are ways of improving access to services, information about services among providers, training, or resource exchange.

Organizational Practices

Organizational practices are process variables which involve the participants in producing the desired outcomes. They are, first, community *participation*. Respondents were asked to report the involvement in a venture, or non-involvement, of twenty-five institutions. They then rated the involvement as providing either central or secondary forms of support. A summary score was constructed of *extensive* or *non-extensive participation* and five submeasures were constructed of participation by institutional sectors (state agencies, public agencies, local voluntary agencies, local governments, and private business groups).

The second measure of practice is called organizational *intensity*. This measure included four components: *complexity* (the number of subgroups in the organization), the *number of meetings* in a venture, the *frequency of meetings*, and *formal records*. The third measure focused on methods of data collection for *needs assessment*. Eleven methods were summed additively (program evaluation, agency records, referral data, feedback from volunteers, Delphi, Force Field Analysis, survey of practitioners, advisory group, interagency exchange data, political consultation, and interagency consultation).

Another practice measure documented sources of *input* from citizens or clients, summed additively (citizens surveyed, citizens in meetings, clients surveyed, clients in meetings). The fifth practice measure attempted to identify the extent to which multiple sources of support were pursued. The measure is called *resource mobilization*. Respondents reported whether any of eleven sources of funding were approached. The eleven sources are federal, city, state, or county governments; business or industry; fund-raising events; memberships; United Way; individual contributors; and loans of personnel, or exchange of materials or facilities. These items were then summed additively to construct a multiple resource score.

Finally, a measure was constructed on resource *negotiating strategies*: using new resources, shifting existing resources, or pulling resources together, summed additively.

Outcome

The outcome variable is *effectiveness*, a subjective measure of the success of the planning venture as identified by respondents. They were asked simply to evaluate whether they were highly successful, moderately successful, or not at all successful in achieving their goals.

These measures are the basis of the following analysis of data.

FINDINGS

Urban-Rural Differences

No difference between urban and rural areas is found in organizational form. Mandated and voluntary organizations are just as prevalent in each area. In the case of goals, however, a clear difference is found. Rural areas tend to focus on direct service goals whereas urban areas show higher rates of procedural goal setting (see Table 1). For example, urban areas were more likely to report that they were working on interagency channels of communication or exchange on behalf of client services.

Greater rural-urban differences are found in organizational practices. Urban areas show much more extensive participation across community institutions. Similarly, organizational intensity is much higher in urban areas. Attempts to leverage various public and private resources occur more frequently in urban areas and efforts to

Table 1: Urban-Rural Differences

	Gamma	Kendall's Tau	Significance
Goals	0.37	0.23	0.041
Participation	0.68	0.65	0.000
Intensity	0.48	0.46	0.002
Needs Assessment	0.52	0.49	0.001
Resource Mobilization	0.55	0.43	0.006
Resource Negotiations	0.27	0.18	0.05

exchange resources between leverage points occur more often in urban areas.

Urban areas favored the tougher negotiating strategies of developing new resources or shifting resources. The relatively benign strategy of "pulling resources together" appears to fit the environmental requirements of rural areas better than the strategy of "using new resources." This finding makes sense when viewed in light of the relative scarcity of available talent and wealth in the rural areas for obtaining new resources. Perhaps the strategy of pulling resources together fits better the networking talents of the small community. Further research on this point is warranted.

Characteristics of Mandated and Voluntary Organizations

Community planning organizations are characterized as bureaucratically mandated or voluntary. Management teams, legislated boards, and multi-agency staff groups are described as mandated. The participants, who may behave formally or informally, clearly participate as representatives of formal organizations. Networks and councils are viewed here as voluntary. It is assumed that their participants are relatively free to represent the community at large. The data reveal no difference between rural and urban communities in the occurrence of these different types. A comparison of the two types revealed the organizational characteristics listed in Table 2.

Voluntary and mandated organizations do not differ significantly

Table 2: Characteristics of Mandated and Voluntary Organizations

	Gamma	Kendall's Tau	Significance
Goals	0.18	0.08	0.17
Participation	0.08	0.06	0.28
Intensity	0.18	0.11	0.30
Needs Assessment	0.18	0.11	0.11
Input Strategies	0.37	0.26	0.0003
Resource Mobilization	0.13	0.09	0.003
Resource Negotiation	0.13	0.09	0.17
Local Voluntary Participation	0.27	0.20	0.02
Private Participation	0.42	0.31	0.0007

by goals, institutional participation, organizational intensity, needs assessment tools, the number of resource mobilization points, and negotiating strategies. However, voluntary organizations leveraged a greater variety of resources. Mandated groups tended to restrict themselves to one or two sources of funding.

Voluntary organizations employed a greater variety of citizen and client input strategies; mandated groups tended to avoid such input. Two specific categories of institutional participation differed significantly: participation among local voluntary organizations and among private institutions occurred more frequently among voluntary planning organizations. The other categories of institutional participation, state-local agencies, local public agencies, and local governments did not differ significantly.

These findings are suggestive of a pattern of bureaucratic pinpointing among the mandated planning groups and broader based strategies by the voluntary organizations. Bureaucratically mandated planning organizations may have been more narrowly focused while voluntary groups formulated broad based strategies. These findings are not consistent across all measures, but they raise the question of a strategic pattern of organizing which bears further investigation.

In other words, it may be that mandated community planning organizations are more likely than voluntary organizations to follow a path of pinpointed participation, lower intensity of meetings, a narrower range of data collections for needs assessment, pinpointed resource mobilization, and simpler negotiating strategies in order to achieve their objectives. Voluntary organizations, conversely, may be more likely to exhibit broader based organizational practices.

Strategic Patterns of Organizing

The suggestion of strategic organizing patterns raises the question of consistency among the organizational practices. Indeed, extensiveness of institutional participation is correlated with organizational intensity (R = 0.21; Sig = 0.008). Planning organizations which include a broad range of institutional participants also maintain more subcommittees, hold more meetings, meet more frequently, and formalize their records more often than do organizations with a narrow range of institutional participants.

Extensiveness of institutional participation correlates also with mobilizing multiple resource points (R = 0.17; Sig = 0.02); a variety of needs assessment data collection methods (R = 0.23; Sig = 0.005); and a variety of citizen and client input strategies (R = 0.21; Sig = 0.007). These observations leave the impression of an internally related cluster of broad based organizational practices vs. an internally related set of pinpointed practices. A broad based strategic pattern of organizing emerges with extensive and intensive participation, multiple forms of needs assessment and client input, and multiple resource points. In contrast, we find a pinpointing pattern of practices which appear to be related to each other. (See Figure 1).

Effectiveness

The subjective measure of effectiveness must be interpreted cautiously because it is prone to varying interpretations. The respondents, again, were persons identified as contact persons representing their organization. Respondents were asked to evaluate their achievement as "highly successful," "moderately successful," or "not at all" successful. For whatever it is worth, some minor correlations can be reported. The measure of effectiveness correlates with organizational form (mandated vs. voluntary planning organizations), voluntary organizations reporting higher levels of effectiveness (see Table 3). Effectiveness correlates mildly with multiple resource negotiating strategies, type of goal (direct service), and the number of meetings held in a planning venture, though not their frequency. This latter observation is consistent with a finding by Gamson in his historic study, *Strategies of Social Conflict* (Gamson, 1975) which correlated influence over public policies with persistence, as demonstrated by the length of a campaign.

Figure 1

STRATEGIC PATTERNS OF ORGANIZING		
STEPS IN ORGANIZING	PINPOINTED	BROAD-BASED
Organizational form	Mandated	Voluntary
Participation	Narrow	Extensive
Goals	Direct Service	Procedural or both
Intensity	Low	Persistent
Need assessments	Minimal data	Multiple forms of data
Inputs	Minimal	Extensive
Resource mobilization	Few sources of support attempted	Many sources of support attempted
Negotiations	Simple: developing new resources or pulling	Multiple: shifting, developing new resource

Table 3: Effectiveness and Organizational Characteristics

	Gamma	Kendall's Tau	Significance
Goals	0.25	0.15	0.05
Organizational form	0.23	0.14	0.06
Participation	0.13	0.08	0.19
Intensity	0.08	0.03	0.32
Needs Assessment	0.05	0.03	0.35
Input	0.06	0.03	0.35
Resource Mobilization	0.02	0.01	0.43
Resource Negotiations	0.30	0.16	0.03
Number of meetings	0.24	0.14	0.06

Correlation with the subtypes of institutional participation are suggestive. Reports of success occurred more frequently in ventures which included businesses as participants (R = 0.18; Sig = 0.05). Rates of success were lower among ventures which included state-local agencies (R = 0.21; Sig = 0.02). Those agencies are the public welfare agency, youth or court services, and rehabilitative services. Local public agencies also correlated with lower rates of success (R = 0.25; Sig = 0.007). Those are the community action agency, the school system, and services to the aged. These findings are difficult to interpret; it may be that ventures including public agencies face more intractable problems than those involving private businesses. There are fewer resources to accomplish their objectives, and there is less likely to be an optimism and enthusiasm for change.

Most important, the measures of participation, organizational intensity, multiple resource mobilizing points, and varieties of data collection for needs assessment as well as citizen and client input did not correlate with effectiveness.

DISCUSSION

Empirical Findings

Because of the nature of the sample and measures, the findings must be viewed as exploratory. There are four types of measure in this study: (1) community size, which is contextual, (2) the initiating variables, organizational form and goal, (3) organizational practices, and 4) the outcome measure, effectiveness. The correlations reported above among the organizational practices suggests the existence of syndromes: the broad based and pinpointing syndromes. The correlations of the bureaucratically mandated groups with pieces of the pinpointing syndrome suggest a strategic pattern. This pattern provides a way of conserving energy and going, as much as possible, straight to the resource "well" without "wasting" energy. The voluntary groups, on the other hand, may follow the community minded strategy of "covering all bases," looking under every rock, avoiding all possible pitfalls or obstacles, documenting the need for resources, and garnering community wide support to provide resources as a means of ensuring continuing support.

Community size is a different matter. The resource environment of small communities is too sparse to allow the broad based practices to be documented even if it is practiced. Many of the twenty-five institutions involved in the participation score are nonexistent in rural communities. Business involvement is unlikely because a critical mass of discretionary wealth does not exist. People with the time and talent to perform all of the data collection and input technologies do not exist. For these reasons, community minded, energetic efforts may occur in rural communities which do not show up in the data. In fact, the voluntary organizational forms do occur just as frequently in rural areas as in urban areas. They apparently do not, however, have the human and technical resources to pursue additional resources. Because of this, they pursue the negotiating strategy of "pulling resources together" more often than using new resources or shifting resources. Pulling resources together is a cooperative strategy but also a "path of least resistance."

The measure of effectiveness is subjective. Nevertheless, it is interesting that no significant difference is found between effectiveness and urban and rural communities nor between effectiveness and most of the organizational practices. For example, effectiveness does not correlate with participation, intensity, needs assessment practices, input strategies, nor resource mobilization. On the other hand, groups with direct service goals appear to be more effective. Networking groups are more effective. Groups which indicated more than one way of negotiating resources are more effective. Groups meeting over a longer period of time are more effective; and ventures not including a range of public agencies were more effective. Undoubtedly, direct service goals are more inherently motivating, more fundable, and produce fewer interorganizational obstacles than procedural goals.

Theory

With its focus on resources in its heuristic definition of planning, this study is suggestive of an ecological perspective on community organizing. The resource environment of the community has had an evident effect on organizational practices. Communities with some wealth in income and talent expended their wealth in organizational efforts and knowledge based practices. The broad based organizing syndrome, which requires high levels of energy, does not correlate with the measure of effectiveness because a powerful resource environment requires correspondingly higher powered efforts to mobilize a change.

That direct service goals are more effective than procedural goals suggests a strategy of penetrating vertically through the resource environment external to the community. However, the issue of devising a pinpointed strategy vs. broad based involvement is clouded in this study because different ways of formulating a broad based strategy were not considered. For example, the study does not differentiate between "grass roots" and elite strategies. It does not probe the effect of involvement of institutions outside a functional specialty. Do they muddy the waters or do they lend greater credibility to an effort? Further study of these questions is warranted.

Further research is also warranted on the broad based and pinpointing syndromes. Ecological theory focuses on the availability of resources and energy to sustain an "organism" and its activities. Many community organization and planning objectives may justify a "low energy" organizing strategy by virtue of its efficacy in achieving objectives. Such a choice may frequently be justified as a matter of setting human resource priorities among organizing campaigns. The "high energy" option is simply not available to each and every organizing campaign which might be deemed worthy of the attention. The advantages of both the broad based and the pinpointed organizing syndromes, therefore, need to be further documented and analyzed.

Methodology

Two key problems are found in the methodology that can be corrected in similar studies. First, the sample is incomplete largely because of a lack of resources and time to follow up on non-responses. Indeed, with sufficient resources it would have been preferable to spend time networking in each non-responsive county to search for unreported planning organizations and unreturned forms. It is estimated that the sample would have improved from its 67% level of return to over 80% in just one month of full-time work. The sample produces an urban bias, which may in effect underemphasize the differences between the rural and urban communities.

Second, the major defect among the measures is the outcome measure, effectiveness. An approach such as Goal Attainment Scaling might have been more useful in documenting and quantifying the results of a planning venture. In such an approach, the respondent would be asked to state a measurable goal for mobilization of resources, state whether the requisite resources were obtained and the level of adequacy of those resources. This approach emphasizes the process goals of obtaining resources. It is consistent with the ecological perspective and allows relatively meaningful short term measures to be devised. It is also more specific than the vague notion of "success" in achieving goals, thereby yielding less subjective responses. Such a measure would be readily understandable to respondents and relatively easy to document.

A more complex methodology is recommended which requires major resources, assuming large grants are available. To achieve a higher level of reliability of measures, respondents would be treated as informants, as though each measure were the subject of an ethnographic study. A variety of perhaps three different types of informant would be required for each planning organization and each venture: a central leader, a recording secretary, and a marginal member of the group. A degree of consensus would be required for each single measure to be considered reliable. MacNair (1970) developed this methodology in his research on civil rights organizational networks.

CONCLUSIONS

It is the contention of this researcher that the simpler methodology demonstrated in this study achieves a "satisficing" level of reliability for exploratory purposes. Ironically, it may be the more ethnographic approach which achieves a higher level of reliability. In either case, similar forms of survey research can and should be done if a solid and respectable body of knowledge on community interventive practices is to be developed.

The overall findings of this study support the assumption of ecological theory that the resource environment has an appreciable effect on the organizing strategies of community planning organizations. Urban environments afford greater talent in human resources and greater wealth. Organizational practices are correspondingly broader based in urban than in rural areas. Participation across institutions is much more extensive in urban communities; meetings are more intensive; greater variety of inputs are included in needs assessments; more extensive forms of resource mobilization are utilized; and tougher resource negotiation strategies are attempted. The irony in this study is that these higher energy, broad based practices do not produce greater subjective effectiveness, given the nature of goals being pursued. In the urban environment, goals are more likely to be procedural and interorganizational than in the rural environment where goals are more likely to be focused on developing direct services. In the resource starved environment of rural communities we find, then, an energy conserving, pinpointed organizing strategy which is focused clearly on the development of direct services. In the relatively rich environment of urban communities we find a high energy, broad based organizing strategy which struggles to achieve its objectives among high powered bureaucratic structures.

Compounding this picture is the serendipitous finding that ventures among private and voluntary institutions are more likely to be deemed effective. Public agencies face more intractable problems, I assume, and are less likely to achieve the cooperation and the resources they need to meet their goals.

This study cannot document the greater effectiveness of either the conservative pinpointed organizing syndrome or the higher powered, broad based sets of organizational practices. It suggests, however, that the greater the hurdle the greater is the likelihood of using the higher powered organizing strategies. It follows that networking organizations or voluntary councils are more likely the structures of choice, with their presumed community-mindedness, as opposed to mandated commissions or management teams. Further research is needed to document the conditions that warrant a conservative "satisficing" strategic pattern of organizing and those conditions which require an "all out" broad based strategy.

One other unexpected finding is suggestive. The number of meetings in a venture, not the intensity or frequency of meetings, correlates with effectiveness. It may be that long-term persistence is more important than short-term, "frenetic" activity.

It is not suggested that a practitioner should follow one or the other set of patterns slavishly. A professional, "ecological" practitioner will assess the environment for the availability of resources for organizing the entire planning process in order to design a feasible strategic organizing pattern. Such a practitioner will re-assess organizing resources at each step of the organizing process. Each element of the strategy may be designed in pinpointed fashion or broad based fashion, depending on the critical need to demonstrate clout as well as the availability of organizing talent and funds.

REFERENCES

Agar, M. *Speaking of ethnography*. Newbury Park, CA: Sage, 1986.

Blakely, E. *Planning local economic development: Theory and practice*. Newbury Park: CA: Sage, 1989.

Brager, G., Specht, H. & Torczyner, J. *Community organizing* (2nd ed.). New York: Columbia University Press, 1987.

Callahan, J. Obstacles and Social Planning, *Social Work*, 1973, *18*, 70-79.

Cox, F. et al. *Tactics and techniques of community practice*. Itasca, IL: F.E. Peacock, 1977.

Cummings, S. & Glaser, M. Neighborhood participation in community development: a comparison of strategic approaches, *Population Research and Policy Review*, 1985, *4*, 267-287.

Deseran, F. Community development and images of influence structures: some conceptual and methodological considerations. *Journal of the community development society*, 1980, *11*, 23-34.

Ecklein, J. & Lauffer, A. *Community organizers and social planners*. New York: Wiley and Sons, 1971.

Ecklein, J. *Community Organizers*. New York: Wiley and Sons, 1983.

Fellin, P. *The community and the social worker*. Itasca, New York: Peacock, 1987.

Fielding, N., & Fielding, J. *Linking data*. Newbury Park, CA: Sage, 1986.

Gamson, W. *The strategy of social protest*. Homewood, IL: Dorsey Press, 1975.

Glaser, B. & Strauss, A. *The discovery of grounded theory*. Chicago: Aldine-Atherton Press, 1967.

Hawley, A. *Human ecology: A theory of community structure*. New York: Ronald Press, 1950.

Holland, T. The community: Organism or arena. *Social Work*, 1974, *19*, 73-80.

Hughes, J. & Mann, L. Systems and planning theory. *Journal of the American Institute of Planners*, 1969, *35*, 330-333.

Kramer, R. Organization of a community action program: A comparative case study. *Social Work*, 1967, *12*, 68-80.

Lauffer, A. *Assessment tools: for practitioners, managers, and trainers*. Beverly Hills: Sage, 1982.

Lauffer, A. *Getting the resources you need*. Beverly Hills: Sage, 1982.

Lauffer, A. *Social planning at the community level.* Englewood Cliffs, NJ: Prentice-Hall, 1978.

Leiter, M. & Webb, M. *Developing human services networks.* New York: Irvington Publishers, 1983.

Long, N. *The unwalled city: Reconstituting the urban community,* New York: Basic Books, 1972.

MacNair, R. *Civil rights organizational networks in Cleveland, Ohio, and Birmingham, Alabama: A study of kin organizations.* Unpublished doctoral dissertation, University of Michigan, 1970.

MacNair, R. Citizen participation in public agencies: Foul Weather Friends. *Administration and Society,* 1983, *14,* 507-524.

Martin, R. *Decisions in Syracuse.* Bloomington, IN: Indiana University Press, 1962.

Meenaghan, T. *Macro practice in social work.* New York: Free Press, 1982.

McKillup, J. *Need analysis: Tools for the human services and education.* Newbury Park, CA: Sage, 1987.

Melvin, P. *The organic city: Urban definition and neighborhood organization, 1880-1920.* Lexington, KY: University of Kentucky Press, 1987.

Neuber, K. *Needs assessment: A model for community planning.* Beverly Hills, CA: Sage, 1980.

Orden, S. The impact of community action programs on private social service agencies. *Social Problems,* 1973, *20,* 364-381.

Rothman, J. *Planning and organizing for social change: Action principles from social science research.* New York: Columbia University Press, 1974.

Rothman, J. & Erlich, J. *Promoting innovation and change in organizations and communities: A planning manual.* New York: John Wiley and Sons, 1976.

Rubin, H. & Rubin I. *Community organizing and development.* Columbus, OH: C.E. Merrill, 1986.

Shostak, A. Promoting participation of the poor: Philadelphia's antipoverty program. *Social Work,* 1966, *11,* 64-72.

Suttles, G. *The social order of the slum: Ethnicity and territory in the inner city.* Chicago: The University of Chicago Press, 1968.

Taylor, S. & Roberts, R. *Theory and practice of community social work.* New York: Columbia University Press, 1985.

Tropman, J. Comparative analysis of community organization agencies: The case of the welfare council. In I.A. Spergel (Ed.), *Community organization: Studies in constraint.* Beverly Hills: Sage, 1972.

Verma, S. Effectiveness of advisory committees in community resource development. *Journal of the Community Development Society,* 1986, *17,* 41-54.

Warren, R. Application of social science knowledge to the community organization field. *Journal of Education for Social Work,* 1967, *3,* 60-72.

Warren, R., Rose, S., & Bergrunder, A. *The structure of urban reform.* Lexington, MA: Lexington Books, 1974.

Waste, R. *The ecology of city policy making.* New York: Oxford University Press, 1989.

Strategic Choices Made
by Nonprofit Agencies
Serving Low-Paying Clients

Steven L. McMurtry, PhD
Peter M. Kettner, DSW
F. Ellen Netting, PhD

INTRODUCTION

For administrators of nonprofit human service agencies, the
1980s was a decade in which each new fiscal year brought fewer
resources than necessary to maintain services at existing levels. A
major cause of this problem was declining public revenues, evidenced by the 35% reduction in inflation-adjusted federal spending
for social welfare programs in just the two-year span from 1980 to
1982 (Salamon & Abramson, 1982). Also, though charitable contributions grew during the early part of the decade, social service
agencies' share of these funds declined (Hodgkinson & Weitzman,
1986). The effect of these changes was to force social work administrators to spend a considerable amount of time and energy on planning, preparing, and, all too often, cutting back their agency's budget.

Devising rational means to address budgetary problems is a subject that has interested organizational writers for many years. Program and functional budgeting techniques have been designed to

Dr. McMurtry is Assistant Professor, Dr. Kettner is Professor, and Dr. Netting
is Associate Professor, School of Social Work, Arizona State University, Tempe,
AZ 85287.

An earlier version of this article was presented at the Annual Program Meeting
of the Council on Social Work Education, Reno, Nevada, 1990.

permit an increase or decrease in the volume of services based on available revenues (Lee & Johnson, 1973). Zero-based budgeting, while never gaining wide acceptance as a comprehensive budgeting method, left behind some useful concepts such as the organizing of budget-related "decision packages" designed to facilitate rational approaches to budgeting (Pyhrr, 1973).

More specifically connected to the voluntary sector, Vinter and Kish (1984) proposed an approach to making budget-cutting decisions that is tailored to human service agencies. In this model the planner divides expenses into immediate, proximate, and distant categories, with expenses involving direct services to clients being considered the most immediate. Items in the immediate category would receive the highest priority for retention of funding; those in the distant category would be the first candidates for budget reductions.

One shortcoming of the above approaches is that they focus on decision making that is largely based on factors internal to the agency. In so doing, they ignore the extreme vulnerability of most agencies to external forces in their organizational environments. As trends in the 1980s have demonstrated, these environments are often turbulent and unpredictable.

This article reports on results of a study designed to examine how private, nonprofit human service agencies responded to environmental changes during the late 1980s. One phase of the study addressed the hypothesis that the order in which nonprofit agencies employed adaptive strategies would conform to a theoretical model. In addition, the study sought to determine whether certain types of environmental changes were associated with specific actions on the part of these agencies. Particular attention was directed toward agencies that serve clients who are able to pay little or nothing for their services in order to determine whether these clients are disproportionally affected by the choice of certain strategies.

ENVIRONMENTAL CHANGES AS DETERMINANTS OF ORGANIZATIONAL ACTIONS

Though a number of classic works in organizational theory address the issue of how agencies maintain themselves in such environments, one especially useful piece is James Thompson's 1967 work, *Organizations in Action*. Thompson begins not with a prescription for budgetary decision making but with a prediction about how organizations will behave under conditions of environmental uncertainty. Based on the open-systems model, he suggests that agencies' actions represent attempts to make rational choices among possible responses, beginning with those least disruptive to internal operations and output goals and ending with more drastic measures necessary to ensure organizational survival.

The first set of strategies involves responses designed to *protect the organization's technical core* — its essential production components. These responses begin with efforts to draw on what Thompson calls "technological slack" or unused productive capacity that can be employed to absorb minor variations in an organization's environment without having to change its basic input/output balance. When this slack capacity is exhausted, more active responses to protect the technical core are used, including activities to maintain revenue and client flow and to ensure capacity to remain within the budget. Bozeman and Slusher (1979) call attention to these patterns in their analysis of the behavior of public agencies in times of resource scarcity. They argue that organizations in these circumstances will seek "to maximize the productive capacity of the technology" in order to minimize technological slack and thus improve their survivability.

A second set of strategies for dealing with environmental change comes under the heading of *acquiring power over the environment*. Lacking the ability to absorb environmental changes internally, agencies attempt to manipulate external relationships in order to insure their ability to garner necessary resources from other organizations. The most important such organizations comprise what Pfeffer and Salancik (1978) term the "enacted environment," and members of this group will be the prime focus of an agency's strategic efforts. Example of these efforts include attempts to gain prestige, to keep resource alternatives open, to acquire power over important organizations, or to cooperate with other agencies seeking similar resources.

The third and final set of strategies has to do with *altering the organization's domain*. In relatively stable and predictable environments, organizations seek to achieve what Levine and White (1961) term "domain consensus," in which an agency's boundaries (e.g., its range of services and clients) are established in the course of exchanges with other organizations. In environments characterized by uncertainty or chronic scarcity, however, organizations may be forced to adopt riskier strategies that involve venturing out of their traditional domains, often by broadening operations to incorporate tasks previously performed by others. These strategies can result in changes such as altering clientele, altering the type of services provided to the same clients, or altering geographical boundaries. Other agencies may undertake domain change by merging with a larger organization or by bringing other agencies together under the umbrella of franchise relationships.

Thompson's work focuses primarily on organizations in the commercial sector, and some of his propositions do not fully reflect circumstances in nonprofit agencies. In an earlier work, the authors explored ways in which his assumptions about organizational decision-making priorities can be adapted to human service agencies (McMurtry, Netting & Kettner, 1990). This involves dividing Thompson's initial category of actions to protect the technical core into four subsets: (1) strategies to enhance productivity; (2) strategies to increase revenues; (3) strategies to employ excess or "slack" resources within the organization, and (4) "cutback" strategies — those that are designed to control output by reducing services. Thompson's second major category, strategies to gain power within the agency's "task environment," remains unchanged when applied to human service agencies. The final category, strategies to alter the organization's domain, is termed "restructuring strategies" in the revised model. This reflects the fact that, for nonprofit organizations, all of these actions involve changing the fundamental structure of the agency in some way.

Thompson's proposed ordering of responses is also adjusted in this revised model. Specifically, it is hypothesized that the sequence in which nonprofit agencies employ the above adaptation strategies is as follows:

1. Strategies to enhance productivity (e.g., increase staff training);
2. Strategies to increase revenues (e.g., organize special fundraising events);

3. Strategies to utilize organizational slack (e.g., increase staff caseloads);
4. Strategies to acquire power over the task environment (e.g., join a lobbying coalition);
5. Strategies involving service cutbacks (e.g., turn away service applicants);
6. Strategies to restructure the agency (e.g., merge with another agency).

Table 1 provides additional examples of specific actions that fall within each of these categories.[1]

The above ordering takes the form of a Guttman scale in which there is a descending frequency of use of strategies across categories (Guttman, 1944). If this hypothesis reflects reality, restructuring strategies will be used least frequently, and only when all other categories of strategies have previously been attempted. Similarly, cutback strategies will be used only when the first four categories have been tried, and so on. The distinguishing characteristic of this model is that strategies to utilize organizational slack and cutback strategies are both expected to occur later in the sequence than would be inferred from Thompson's original model. This change reflects the authors' view that strategies to utilize organizational slack in human service agencies often involve steps such as freezing new hiring or increasing staff workloads. These actions may come at the expense of staff discontent and thus are likely to be seen as more costly to the agency than efforts to increase productivity or revenues. Since they are presumably contrary to agencies' charitable missions, cutback strategies are expected to be employed only when an agency has tried all other responses short of substantially restructuring itself.

METHODOLOGY

The study instrument was an eight-page written questionnaire mailed to the chief administrator of each of 440 human service agencies in the state of Arizona. These agencies were sampled from an initial list of more than 1,400 organizations included in an information and referral directory covering human service providers in 12 of the 15 counties in the state. One urban county, encompassing

TABLE 1

Strategies Most Commonly Used to Respond to
Environmental Changes (n = 167)

Strategy	Percent Using Strategy
Strategies to Increase Productivity	
1. Initiate efforts to improve coordination of and mutual problem-solving by staff	92.6
2. Increase employee participation in decision making	91.1
3. Increase staff recognition and/or implement productivity inducements	85.2
4. Initiate or increase staff training efforts	85.1
Strategies to Increase Revenues	
1. Appeal to new funding sources	83.5
2. Conduct special fundraising efforts	80.6
3. Increase efforts to gain media attention in order to increase charitable donations	78.8
4. Increase board members' participation in fundraising	78.4
Strategies to Utilize Organizational "Slack"	
1. Rely more heavily on volunteers	76.0
2. Increase staff workloads	73.0
3. Computerize record keeping to increase efficiency and reduce personnel costs	69.7
4. Limit overtime/compensatory time	58.5
Strategies to Acquire Power Over the Task Environment	
1. Expand networking with other agencies to increase the agency's power and influence	88.4
2. Restructure board composition to increase the agency's power and influence	74.6
3. Increase time spent making legislative contacts	61.0
4. Join a voluntary association for lobbying and unified action	58.6
Strategies Involving Service Cutbacks	
1. Provide services on a first-come, first-served basis until resources are exhausted	51.1
2. Eliminate or shrink programs	51.0
3. Increase waiting time between application and receipt of services	38.0
4. Reduce outreach	37.4

Strategies to Restructure the Organization

1.	Merge with other organization(s)	28.3
2.	Consider terminating the agency	25.0
3.	Franchise one or more of your programs	18.4
4.	Become a franchise of a larger organization	17.5

the Phoenix metropolitan area, accounted for about half the agencies on the list; the other half were distributed among the remaining 11 rural counties.

Criteria used to define nonprofit human service agencies included the following: (1) incorporation as a private, nonprofit organization (under Section 501(c)(3) of the Internal Revenue Service codes); (2) presence of a formal structure and budget; (3) employment of professional or volunteer staff; and (4) having a primary function of providing services to clients who were not members of the organization. Organizations that did not meet these criteria were removed from the list of potential survey recipients. Among those removed were voluntary membership organizations (such as service clubs and scout groups), as well as hospitals and other primary-care health providers.[2] The remaining agencies reflected the diversity that exists among human service organizations, from food banks to family counseling centers and from small-scale rural providers to multi-office metropolitan affiliates of national organizations.

The elimination process decreased the original list to 960 agencies, from which 440 were randomly chosen to receive the questionnaire. Forty-seven agencies for which mailings were undeliverable or that were found not to qualify as non-profit service organizations were discarded from the sample, leaving 393 valid agencies. Completed questionnaires were received from 198 of these, giving a final response rate of 50.4%.

Respondents were asked to indicate whether their agency served clients from each of the following groups: (1) clients who paid as much or more as the break-even cost of the service (either personally or via a third party); (2) clients whose service costs were covered by purchase-of-service contracts; and (3) clients who paid less than the break-even cost of services (including those who paid nothing at all). As noted earlier, the focus of this article is on the third and last group, thus the results reported below are based on the 167 agencies (84.3%) that reported serving at least some low-pay clients.

RESULTS

Frequency and Sequential Ordering of Response Types

Each questionnaire presented a list of strategic responses organized according to the categories identified in the hypothesis. Respondents were asked to indicate all strategies that their agency had employed during the previous three fiscal years. Table 1 displays the four most commonly reported strategies in each category. A quick visual review of the table indicates that the frequency of use of strategies across categories generally conforms to the hypothesis. For example, productivity-enhancement strategies were the most common, with the top four strategies in this category being used more frequently than those in any other category. Similarly, four of the five strategies that were next most commonly used were in the revenue-enhancement category. Also as expected, the four least common responses fell into the category of restructuring strategies, and cutback strategies were next in order of those least commonly used.

Tests of whether the ordering of responses conformed to Guttman scaling were conducted via the computation of three statistics — the coefficient of reproducibility (CR), the coefficient of scalability (CS), and minimum marginal reproducibility (MMR). The first two, CR and CS, address the degree to which response patterns correspond to a theoretical ideal, each providing a different measure of the goodness of fit between observed and expected scores. MMR is used primarily as a check for CR, which is susceptible to distortion by extreme marginal distributions. The convention used by most researchers in interpreting these values is that CR must be .90 or more, MMR must be less than .90 (the farther below CR the better), and CS must be .60 or more (McIver & Carmines, 1981). Values for these statistics were obtained via the GUTTMAN procedure in the SAS computer package (SAS Institute, 1986).

Six variables were created for the analysis. Each variable was a dummy-coded indicator of whether any strategy from each of the six response categories was employed by a given agency. The percentage of agencies using at least one strategy from each of the six categories was as follows:

- Strategies to enhance productivity — 86.8%
- Strategies to increase revenues — 95.7%
- Strategies to utilize organizational slack — 85.6%
- Strategies to acquire power over the task environment — 83.2%
- Strategies involving service cutbacks — 41.3%
- Strategies to restructure the agency — 34.1%.

Table 2 shows the results of tests on three different models. Findings from the test of the first model, which included all six categories of strategies, indicate that this sequence of variables did not scale as hypothesized (due to a CS value less than .60). One prob-

TABLE 2

Scalability of Hierarchical Models

Variables*	N	CR	MMR	CS
Model 1				
Pro - Rev - Sla - Pow - Cut - Res	138	.90	.80	.51
Model 2				
Pro - Sla - Pow - Cut - Res	167	.90	.76	.58
Model 3				
Pro/Sla - Pow - Cut - Res	167	.90	.74	.60

```
* Key to abbreviations:
    Pro - Productivity-enhancement strategies
    Rev - Revenue-enhancement strategies
    Sla - Slack-utilization strategies
    Pow - Power-enhancement strategies
    Cut - Cutback strategies
    Res - Restructuring strategies
    Pro/Sla - Combined slack/productivity variable
```

lem with this model, however, was that the variable indicating the use of revenue-enhancement strategies contained a number of missing values. The next model therefore excluded the revenue-enhancement variable so that the remaining responses could be tested on all 167 agencies. This model also failed to meet the scaling criteria, again because of a CS value below .60.

In order better to understand these results, the authors analyzed zero-order correlations among the remaining variables. This revealed a relatively high correlation ($r = .69$) between productivity-enhancement strategies and slack-utilization strategies. Based on this finding, a final model was constructed in which a new variable was computed to indicate whether an agency had used *either* productivity-enhancement or slack-utilization strategies. As shown in Table 2, this final model met the criteria for scalability across all three coefficients. This suggests that agencies do follow a hierarchy of responses to environmental changes in a sequence that (1) begins with productivity-enhancement and/or slack-utilization strategies, (2) proceeds to power-enhancement strategies, (3) employs cutback strategies, and (4) culminates with efforts to restructure the agency.

Correlates of Strategic Choice

In addition to analyzing the range and ordering of strategic choices among non-profit providers, the study also sought to begin the process of determining the conditions under which particular choices are made. Specifically, the authors set out to explore whether strategic choices, especially those involving service cutbacks, were associated with changes in revenue, changes in interagency competition (e.g., for clients or revenues), or changes in service demand. Previous works have posited that service cutbacks are most likely to occur when revenues drop (due to increased competition or decreased availability of funding) or when demand for services to low-pay clients is on the rise (Coulton, Rosenburg, & Yankey, 1981; McMurtry, Netting & Kettner, 1990). Low-pay clients usually bear the brunt of such cuts precisely because they do not provide revenues to offset the cost of their services.

In this survey, each agency was asked to indicate trends it had experienced during the previous three fiscal years in: (1) demand for services coming from low-pay clients; (2) availability of revenues to offset the cost of serving these clients; and (3) competition for these revenues from other providers. Results showed that virtually all agencies that served low-pay clients had experienced steady or increasing demand for services from this group and steady or increasing competition for funds to pay for these services. The only trend in which there was analyzable variation among agencies was in the pattern of availability of revenues to offset the cost of serving low-pay clients. Among the responding agencies, 56% reported that these revenues had increased or remained steady during the previous three years, while 44% reported decreases.

Table 3 details the results of a series of bivariate correlations computed between trends in revenues available to serve low-pay clients and the use of strategies from each major category. Revenue trend was coded as decreasing versus steady or increasing, while

TABLE 3

Correlations Between Strategic Choices and Trends in
Revenues for Serving Low-Pay Clients (n = 134)*

Category of Strategy	Use of Any Strategy in the Category		Number of Strategies Used in the Category	
	r	Sig.	r	Sig.
Strategies to Increase Productivity	**	**	-.17	.03
Strategies to Enhance Revenues	**	**	-.10	.12
Strategies to Utilize Organizational Slack	-.12	.07	-.18	.02
Strategies to Acquire Power within the Environment	-.21	.01	-.17	.03
Strategies Involving Service Cutbacks	-.15	.05	-.17	.03
Strategies to Alter the Organizational Domain	-.10	.11	-.04	.29

* Coding for revenue trend is: 0 - Decreasing; 1 - Steady or increasing.
** Insufficient variance to compute correlation coefficient.

the selection of strategies was analyzed as: (1) whether any strategy from each category was employed; and 2) the number of strategies from the category that were used.

The first two columns in the table detail the Pearson's r and corresponding level of significance for the relationship between revenue trends and the use of any strategy from each of the six categories. (Note that for the first two categories of productivity- and revenue-enhancement strategies, every agency used at least one such strategy, thus no variation was available to analyze.) Among the remaining four categories, declining revenues were found to be statistically significantly associated with the use of both power-enhancement and cutback strategies.

Relative to the number of strategies employed from within each category, figures in the second two columns of the table indicate that revenue declines were significantly associated with the use of a greater number of strategies in the productivity-enhancement, slack-utilization, power-enhancement, and service-cutback categories. In short, declining revenue seems to go hand in hand both with efforts to make internal adjustments and with efforts to gain greater control over external revenue sources. However, trends in the availability of revenues were *not* significantly associated with increases or decreases in the use of strategies from the revenue-enhancement category.[3]

DISCUSSION

The results of this study have focused attention on organizational strategies in times of environmental uncertainty. In the following section, we will comment on certain key areas of the results, including the sequencing of risky versus less risky strategies, decisions to employ restructuring strategies, relationships between revenues and strategic choice, and the ubiquity of efforts to expand revenues. We then conclude with a discussion of the implications of these findings.

Before proceeding with this discussion, however, certain limitations of the study should be noted. First, while the sample from which these findings were obtained may be representative of nonprofit human service agencies in Arizona, regional variations in economic conditions, governmental policies, and the structure of the service system mean that agencies in other states may behave somewhat differently. Also, as the descriptive data illustrate, nonprofit agencies vary widely from one to the next, thus strategic responses in a particular individual or group of agencies may also differ substantially from the general patterns reported here. Finally, the authors recognize that strategic decision-making is a complex process in which a vast range of factors may be taken into account. As was noted in reference to the small effect sizes appearing in Table 3, many such factors could not be addressed in this research and remain to be evaluated in future studies.

Delaying Service Cutbacks

Thompson contends that strategies to protect the technical core are an organization's first line of defense against environmental change. These responses are inwardly focused, seeking to make adjustments to operations or structures that fall within the organization's control. In adapting to environmental change, the nonprofit human service agencies in this study conformed in part to Thompson's predictions in that they customarily began with internally oriented responses such as strategies to enhance productivity or utilize organizational slack.

Continuing Thompson's logic, the next step should have been the use of cutbacks—further responses to protect the technical core. However, administrators in this study delayed cutbacks until they had first tried externally-oriented efforts such as seeking to alter power relationships in the task environment. This is a potentially risky course of action, since it extends the agency into a much larger and less controllable arena. However, as hypothesized, nonprofit providers appeared willing to take this risk.

The reason for this shift may be that rationality in selecting strategies entails more considerations than addressed by Thompson, particularly when it comes to the management of nonprofit human service organizations. For example, in a discussion of decision-making processes, Child (1972), notes that "when incorporating strategic choice in a theory of organization, one is recognizing the operation of an essentially political process in which constraints and opportunities are functions of the power exercised by decision makers in the light of ideological values'' (p. 16). In this study, administrators of nonprofit organizations may have been responding to the political process alluded to by Child, as well as to the balance between this process and ideological values.

For example, if serving poor clients is valued as the ideology around which a human service organization functions, then cutting back services to those clients represents a retreat from that administrative responsibility. Even if cutback strategies such as shrinking or eliminating programs allow the agency to stabilize itself in an uncertain environment, administrators of the agencies in this study delayed such actions. Instead, they attempted to maximize alliances with other groups and organizations placing similar value on providing services to vulnerable clients. Power-enhancement strategies, such as networking, demonstrated that these administrators first focused on how they might influence the environment and decision makers external to their agencies *before* they considered the reduction of client services. Theoretically, this is a riskier strategy than continuing to focus on actions that are within the control of the organization, yet ideologically this speaks to the commitment of nonprofit administrators who believe that there is a balance between running a nonprofit as a ''business'' and operating a service agency devoted to meeting human need.

Restructuring Strategies

When strategies to acquire power within the environment failed or were not sufficient, administrators resorted to cutting back services before they acted to restructure their organizations. Only one-third of the respondents reported using restructuring strategies, a finding that supports the expectation that organizations avoid as long as possible any actions that involve altering their basic structure. For example, a typical agency appears more likely to decide to eliminate a program than to merge with another organization. The reason for this is that merging with another organization may mean a loss of identity, changes in staff, loss of decision-making control, and a host of other potential threats. These threats were apparently viewed as a greater risk than the possible consequences of reducing services, including being criticized for ignoring client needs. Still, the results suggest that at least one in three social work administrators can expect to face this type of hard choice—whether to downsize and maintain what is or to alter the fundamental structure of their agencies.

Revenues and Strategic Choice

Relative to correlations between trends in revenues and the use of particular types of strategies, one noteworthy result was the weak but statistically significant association between the availability of funds and the use of cutback strategies. Both the decision to employ cutbacks and the number of these strategies employed were negatively correlated with the availability of funds to pay for service to low-pay clients. This result suggests that, though the agencies responding to the survey did not make service cutbacks a regular part of their strategic repertoire, they nevertheless adopted these measures when faced with the loss of revenues. For example, roughly half of the agencies reported that they had at some time employed at least one type of cutback response.

Of course, the fact that agencies act to ensure their on-going viability even at the cost of service cutbacks does not necessarily mean they are shirking their responsibilities to vulnerable clients. The only predictable aspect of the environment of most nonprofit providers is that it will continue to change, thus an agency that cuts services today may survive to restore them tomorrow when funding opportunities improve. These kinds of conflicts between environmental exigencies and the needs of clients are inherent in decision-making in nonprofit organizations.

Finally, though a clear pattern appeared relative to the order in which most categories of strategies were selected, revenue-enhancement strategies did not follow the expected sequence. Though these actions were among the most common responses to environmental change, they were apparently employed independent of other strategies that were being used. Also, paradoxically, the use of revenue-enhancement strategies was not significantly associated with changes in the availability of funds. Instead, it appears that revenue-seeking efforts are on-going, everyday aspects of agency operations that do not necessarily correlate with environmental fluctuations.

This finding is important in shedding light on the current roles of social work administrators. For example, to the degree that a myth (or hope?) still lingers that boards of directors rather than administrators are primarily responsible for fundraising, these results should help dispel this illusion. Certainly boards of directors engage in fundraising activities, but the vast majority of respondents indicated that they carry out these tasks on a more or less daily basis, and part of their efforts are directed toward getting board members to participate in the process. This means that training in fundraising techniques must be a prominent part of the education of future social work administrators. This also ties in closely with the need for administrators to understand political processes and the nature of the task environment in which they operate.

Implications

One important aspect of the study's results are its implications for the education of future administrators in schools of social work. For example, the finding that administrators delay the use of service cutbacks until they have first attempted to alter power relationships in their environment suggests the hope that service cutbacks may be forestalled by skillful manipulation of environmental relationships. This in turn implies that the development of this skill in administration students should be a significant aspect of their training. For example, Kessler (1987) points out that the ability to choose agencies with which to ally from among the diversity of organizations in a "pluralistic" environment may be critical to success in environmental interactions. To do this, administrators must be skilled in networking and coalition-building, and they must also be able to assess accurately the ideological orientation of potential allies. These are skills that are not typically covered in social work administration courses, yet they may be essential in avoiding service cutbacks.

Similarly, Weinbach (1990) discusses the importance of the task environment in which human service organizations function. Unlike business organizations, human service agencies have multiple constituencies that can either support or oppose organizational goals. "For those human service organizations that lack the good fortune of having a friendly task environment, a social worker's management tasks must be devoted in part to negotiating with the hostile environment in order to improve relationships" (p. 26). Preparing administrators for practice in human service organizations is therefore quite different from preparing persons to manage commercial enterprises. Whereas paying customers will determine whether they desire an organization's product in the for-profit world, nonprofit organizations serve many persons who cannot pay for the services they desire. Administrators do not have to "sell" their products to their consumers. It is external decision makers, the gatekeepers for both public and private sources of funding, who must be convinced that vulnerable clients should be served. Therefore, administrators in nonprofit human service organizations must be skilled in negotiating their way through a politicized environment and in using strategies to acquire power within that environment.

The results of the study are also useful in offering a means of predicting the sequence of agency responses to environmental change and of anticipating the circumstances under which cutbacks are employed. The implications for current and future administrators of nonprofit human services agencies are many. First, fundraising is developing into a daily activity for administrators, and few can expect to rely on boards of directors to perform these functions. Developing and honing skills in these areas will thus be increasingly important, as will skills in locating alternative and often competitive funding sources in a changing environment. Second, traditional management skills involving the ability to maximize productivity and utilize slack resources may be critical to obtaining successful results from initial efforts to accommodate to environmental change. Third, administrators still cannot focus exclusively on internal operations, no matter how skilled they are in matters of personnel, policies, and procedures. To the contrary, the importance of external factors means that human service administrators must continue to hone their skills in dealing with multiple constituencies, networking with other organizations, and understanding political forces in order to successfully obtain necessary resources from their environments. As the sequence of responses suggests, avoidance of service cutbacks may well rest with an administrator's success in analyzing the environment and establishing viable relationships therein.

NOTES

1. For a more complete review of strategic actions employed by nonprofit providers, see McMurtry, Netting & Kettner (1990).

2. Criteria used to define nonprofit human service agencies were adapted from Kramer (1981). Hospitals and other primary-care providers were excluded from the sample due to the traditional distinctions between health care and social services. Membership organizations (what Kramer terms "voluntary associations") were also excluded because their different functions and revenue sources (e.g., membership dues) mean that their responses to environmental changes might be distinct from those of non-membership service agencies.

3. As a cautionary note, it is important to point out that, though statistically significant in many cases, the correlation coefficients in Table 3 are consistently low, meaning that the explanatory power of revenue trends with respect to agencies' choice of strategies is very limited. For example, the largest coefficient, $r = -.21$, expressing the relationship between resource availability and the use of power-enhancement strategies, indicates that variation in the former accounts for only about 4% of variation in the latter (derived by squaring the value of the coefficient).

REFERENCES

Bozeman, B., & Slusher, E.A. Scarcity and environmental stress in public organizations: A conjectural essay. *Administration in Society*, 1979, *11*, 335-355.

Child, J. Organization structure, environment, and performance: The role of strategic choice. *Sociology*, 1972, *6*, 1-22.

Coulton, C.J., Rosenburg, M.L., & Yankey, J.A. Scarcity and the rationing of services. *Public Welfare*, 1981, *39*, 15-21.

Guttman, L.L. A basis for scaling qualitative data. *American Sociological Review*, 1944, *9*, 139-150.

Hodgkinson, V. & Weitzman, M. *Dimensions of the independent sector*. Washington, DC: The Independent Sector, 1986.

Kessler, M. Interorganizational environments, attitudes, and the policy outputs of public agencies: A comparative case study of legal service agencies. *Administration and Society*, 1987, *19*, 48-73.

Kramer, R.M. *Voluntary agencies in the welfare state*. Berkeley: University of California Press, 1981.

Lee, R.D., & Johnson, R.W. *Public budgeting systems*. Baltimore: University Park Press, 1973.

Levine, S. et al. Exchange as a conceptual framework for the study of interorganizational relationships. *Administrative Science Quarterly*, 1961, *5*, 583-601.

McIver, J.P. & Carmines, E.G. *Unidimensional Scaling*. Series on Quantitative Applications in the Social Sciences, No. 24. Beverly Hills: Sage, 1981.

McMurtry, S.L., Netting, F.E. & Kettner, P.M. Critical inputs and strategic choice in non-profit human service agencies. *Administration in Social Work*, 1990, *14*(3), 67-82.

Pfeffer, J. & Salancik, G.R. *The external control of organizations*. New York: Harper & Row, 1978.

Pyhrr, P.A. *Zero-based budgeting: A practical management tool for evaluating expenses*. New York: Wiley Publications, 1973.

SAS Institute. *Supplementary Library User's Guide, Version 5*. Cary, NC: SAS Institute, 1986.

Salamon, L.M. & Abramson, A.J. *The nonprofit sector and the new federal budget*. Washington, DC: The Urban Institute, 1982.

Thompson, J.D. *Organizations in action*. New York: McGraw-Hill, 1967.

Vinter, R.D. & Kish, R.K. *Budgeting for not-for-profit organizations*. New York: The Free Press, 1984.

Weinbach, R. *The social worker as manager: Theory and practice*. New York: Longman, 1990.

PART 3: SUCCESSFUL SOCIAL CHANGE INITIATIVES: CASE STUDIES FROM THE FIELD

Creating Change for Children with Serious Emotional Disorders: A National Strategy

Barbara J. Friesen, PhD

INTRODUCTION

More than 12 percent of children (approximately 7.5 million) in the U.S. have a mental health problem in need of treatment, and about half of those children have problems that are severe and persistent to the extent that they are considered "seriously emotionally disturbed" (National Advisory Mental Health Council, 1990). De-

Dr. Friesen is Professor, Graduate School of Social Work, Portland State University, P.O. Box 751, Portland, OR 97207, and Director, Research & Training Center on Family Support and Children's Mental Health, Regional Research Institute.

This study was supported by a grant from the National Institute on Disability and Rehabilitation Research, U.S. Department of Education and the National Institute of Mental Health, U.S. Department of Health and Human Services (NIDRR Grant Number G0087C0222-88).

An earlier version of the paper was presented at the Association on Community Organization and Social Administration Symposium, Annual Program Meeting, Council on Social Work Education, Chicago, 1989.

spite these needs, it is estimated that only one-half of all children who have mental or emotional disorders receive any services, and fewer receive services that appropriately address their needs and those of their families (Knitzer, 1982, Saxe, Cross & Silverman, 1988).

The focus of this article is on the efforts of a federally funded project to promote the organization at local, state and national levels of parents whose children have serious emotional disorders . The project, called "Families as Allies," is part of the Research and Training Center on Family Support and Children's Mental Health at the Graduate School of Social Work, Portland State University, Portland, Oregon. The organizing activity took place between 1984 and 1989. Because the activities of the Families as Allies project were closely related to other important developments around the country, the background will be briefly described.

THE CHANGE ENVIRONMENT: NATURE AND SCOPE OF ACTIVITY

In 1984, the Child and Adolescent Service System Program (CASSP) of the National Institute of Mental Health (NIMH) in the U.S. Department of Health and Human Services (HHS) was authorized by Congress. This program provides grants to states for the purpose of developing a comprehensive system of care through establishing a focal point for children's mental health, stimulating better planning for children with serious emotional disorders, and improving service coordination among child-serving agencies. In 1986, two other intentions of the program were articulated as specific goals: (1) to include the family as a resource in both service planning and delivery, and (2) to provide a special focus on minority children and youth. Since 1984, the number of state CASSP projects has increased from the original ten to more than 50; by October, 1990 there were projects in all states (Friesen, Griesbach, Jacobs, Katz-Leavy & Olson, 1988; Lourie, 1990).

Also in 1984, NIMH, in cooperation with the National Institute of Disability and Rehabilitation Research (NIDRR), U.S. Department of Education, established a CASSP Technical Assistance Center at Georgetown University, and two research and training centers; these were the Research and Training Center for Children's

Mental Health at the University of South Florida and the Research and Training Center on Family Support and Children's Mental Health at Portland State University in Portland, Oregon. These centers were designed to improve services for children with serious emotional disorders and their families through programs of research, training, and information dissemination, and were intended to work closely with state CASSP programs to promote service system improvement.

To address the CASSP goals, state CASSP projects engaged in a wide variety of activities, including the development of interagency planning and coordinating bodies, investigation of flexible approaches to the design and funding of services, and implementation of efforts to increase the involvement of family members in the planning, implementation and evaluation of services at the case, agency, and system levels. Strategies to increase family participation included the appointment of family members to planning and advisory groups as well as provision of assistance to parents in organizing support and advocacy groups.

The Research and Training Centers and the CASSP Technical Assistance Center also undertook a wide variety of projects, including research designed to track adolescents as they moved out of the children's service system (Silver, Friedman, Duchnowski & Kutash, 1988), conceptualization of the system of care for children (Stroul & Friedman, 1986), development of models of therapeutic case advocacy (Young, 1990), transition (Modrcin, 1989), and family-centered service (Friesen & Koroloff, 1990), as well as a wide variety of training activities. The efforts of the states and the Research and Training and Technical Assistance Centers all contributed to create a climate within which the family support and parent organizing activities of the Families as Allies project at the Portland Center took place.

CHANGE ISSUES:
THE NEED FOR ADVOCACY

Many reasons for the lack of services for children with serious emotional disabilities and their families can be suggested. These include stigma and lack of public understanding of mental illness and related disorders, general cutbacks in social services during this decade, imperfect knowledge about how to address the problems of these children and their families, and lack of coordination and/or turf battles between agencies responsible for providing services. Saxe and his colleagues (1988) suggest that two major factors that limit the provision of needed services to children with serious emotional disorders are the structure of the health care financing system and a lack of coordination among agencies that provide services to children. These authors assert that other explanations such as inadequate research knowledge "are merely symptoms of systemic difficulties in how public policy has failed children" (p. 800).

Although Saxe and his colleagues may be correct in pointing to the structure of financing and lack of interagency coordination as major barriers to appropriate service, these factors are also merely symptoms of public policy failure. This failure has at its root the low priority given to children and children's problems in this society, exacerbated by specific losses in children's mental health services during the 1980s. The explanation for this low priority is essentially political; it reflects the powerlessness of children in general, and the specific lack of focused and articulate advocacy for children who have serious mental or emotional disorders. This lack of specific advocacy has meant that the needs of children with serious emotional disorders are often not addressed equitably in the resource allocation process. Compared to other childhood disability groups these children and their families do not fare well and within the mental health system children's services are not well developed compared to those for adults with mental illness. In many states, for example, families whose children have developmental disabilities are eligible for a variety of family support services such as respite care, cash assistance, or homemaker services, for which families who have children with emotional disorders often do not qualify. When the CASSP program began in 1984, many state departments of mental health did not have even one position assigned to developing and overseeing children's services.

An additional explanation for the low priority given to mental health services for children was the lack of a vocal advocacy movement. Although organizations such as the Association for Retarded Citizens, the National Down Syndrome Congress, the National Alliance for the Mentally Ill and other disability-focused groups had been very successful in increasing resource allocations and improving services for their constituencies, in 1984 there was no parallel national organization of families focusing on services for children and adolescents with serious emotional disorders, and little organization at the local or state level. Neither of the two major national organizations focused on mental health issues (the National Mental Health Association and the National Alliance for the Mentally Ill) had a clear focus on children's issues.

THE FAMILIES AS ALLIES PROJECT

The Families as Allies project was originally proposed as a small curriculum development project designed to provide professionals with skills in working collaboratively with families whose children had serious emotional disorders. After the project was funded, however, both an intensive review of the professional literature (McManus & Friesen, 1986b) and contact with parents around the country suggested that the project needed to focus more directly on the needs of parents for information, support, and systems change. Accordingly, two major objectives of the project became: (1) to learn about the needs of families, and to assess the services available to meet those needs; and (2) to prepare and disseminate information designed to promote parents' increased capacity to advocate effectively for themselves and their children. No objective related to national organizing was articulated at the beginning of the project, at least in part because the federal grant guidelines did not specifically address this activity. Federal and state personnel, as well as parents, however, recognized the importance of a national voice for children with mental or emotional disorders, and the development of such a voice became an implicit long-term project goal, one to which many other project objectives and activities were oriented.

THE ORGANIZING EFFORT

Strategies Shaped by Actors and Events

The overall approach to organizing, although it rarely involved the open conflict often associated with social action, most closely resembles Rothman's (1979) description of the social action approach:

> The social action approach presupposes a disadvantaged segment of the population that needs to be organized, perhaps in alliance with others, in order to make adequate demands on the larger community for increased resources or treatment more in accordance with social justice or democracy. It aims at making basic changes in major institutions or community practices. Social action . . . seeks redistribution of power, resources, or decision-making in the community and/or changing basic policies of formal organizations. (p. 27)

As Rothman points out, however, the models he suggests are ideal, and most practice contains a mixture of goals and tasks across strategies, as well as over time. That was certainly the case in this instance. The organizing task was complex, and the approach employed contained elements of community development and social planning, as well as social action, as described by Rothman. The organizing approach was shaped by three important factors. These were the characteristics of the population of parents involved, the nature of parent organizations, which contain some built-in contradictions, and the fact that much of the organizing activity was supported by parts of "the system" which the social action effort sought to change.

Characteristics of Parents

Although they have in common the problems and stresses associated with meeting the needs of a seriously troubled child, the parents in question represent a wide cross section of socio-economic status, racial and ethnic groups, and political persuasions. Thus, although they may see themselves as "oppressed" in a general sense, they embody a wide range of ideas about what actions might be appropriate. In addition, many family members feel a great deal of stigma; they may blame themselves for their children's problems, and they may also have been held responsible by family members, or in some cases, professionals (Caplan & Hall-McCorquodale, 1985; Dunst & Trivette, 1987). For these reasons, they may be extremely reluctant to be publicly identified as the parent of a child with serious emotional problems, may be unwilling to attend meetings, and may not be able to consider the exposure associated with public testimony or demonstration. Parents are also very dependent on the system for services for their children, many of whom have severe and persistent problems. They may not like what they have, but are afraid to risk losing it. Thus, many parents are willing to organize for the purpose of giving and receiving support, but are initially less able or willing to see themselves as potential advocates.

The Nature of Parent Groups

Self-help and mutual aid groups involving parents of children with disabilities have three major functions: (1) support; (2) education; and (3) advocacy (Hatfield, 1981; Donner & Fine, 1987). Some parent groups also engage in the provision of necessary direct services not provided through the formal service system (Bersani, 1985). This mixture of needs and functions in parent groups makes the organizing task more difficult and calls for a variety of change strategies. The functions are often not compatible within the same parent groups or organization, at least not at the same time and place (Friesen, 1984). Over time, many parent groups experience internal conflict as some members want to engage in advocacy activities, while others, beset by personal and family crisis, need immediate support, information, and problem-solving services.

These different needs are not only characteristic of different parents within the same group, they are also descriptive of the same families at different points in time. For many families, this potential for severe and recurrent crisis is a "normal" part of living with a child who has serious emotional problems (Olson, 1988). Thus, parents' ability to serve as resources to each other may vary over time, and their capacity for sustained and/or predictable participation in change efforts is often seriously limited.

"System" Support for Advocacy Goals: Inherent Tensions

Promoting the formation of parent self-help and advocacy groups came to be accepted and increasingly encouraged by federal, state and local officials within the mental health and education systems, among others. On the one hand, this support brought resources to the organizing effort; on the other, it presented the specter of cooptation, to which parents became increasingly sensitive. At the beginning of the effort, there was an assumption on the part of some professionals that once organized, the parents would be nothing but helpful partners in advocating for goals valued by professionals. As the effort unfolded, the potential for conflict between the objectives of parents and the objectives of professionals became more apparent, as for example, when parents in one state identified residential treatment as a high priority, which was contrary to the state's movement toward community-based, non-institutional treatment. These and other dilemmas associated with attempts by professionals to promote advocacy and social reform are discussed more fully in other works (e.g., Friesen, 1989; Smith & Moses, 1980). Despite some of these difficulties, both the parents and the professionals involved in this change effort preferred collaborative strategies. These forces resulted in a platform of social action goals pursued mostly through cooperative means.

Problem Solving Approach

Project activities directed toward the development of a national voice were necessarily diffuse at the beginning of the project. Although retrospectively, project activities appear to be sequenced and move in logical steps, in practice, the approach was similar to that described by Lindblom (1977) and Lloyd (1978). Each of these authors recognizes the limitations of linear problem solving approaches when the problems to be solved are complex and the means and ends interdependent. Lloyd (1978) advises treating such problems as open-ended, with flexible boundaries, and points out that the process of exploring the problem may affect its character. In this instance, the overall organizing goal was kept in sight, but short-term objectives, strategies and activities were adopted as opportunities arose and as the results of previous activities emerged.

Initially, although it was difficult to formulate a specific long-term strategy, the need for information was apparent. Little was known about parents' concerns, their needs, or their experiences with seeking services for their children. Neither did adequate information exist about the extent to which parents were involved in some form of organized activity such as local self-help, support, or advocacy groups, although existing evidence suggested that most parents were not involved in mutual aid or advocacy organizations. There was little visible leadership among parents at the state level and none apparent nationally.

Discussions with individual parents around the country revealed that many were unhappy with the current state of affairs; some did not like the way they were treated by professionals, and/or by "the system," many felt isolated and frustrated, and most identified large gaps in educational, therapeutic and support services for their children and families. There was also little information about existing resources for families and no way of knowing what opportunities might arise in the future.

Organizing Principles

Given this situation, four general organizing steps were employed: (1) identify existing leadership and interest among individuals and begin to build a sense of community and a shared identity; (2) help community members obtain the necessary information and skills to engage in problem analysis, planning, and action; (3) assist community members to identify common purposes, goals, and action plans; and (4) help community members create an ongoing structure within which to continue organizing and advocacy efforts.

The published literature contains many examples of how each of these steps are applied at the local neighborhood or community level, but there is little guidance about implementation of change goals on a national basis. The literature on social movements contains some principles and examples of attempts to mobilize large numbers of people around common issues (e.g., Klandermans & Oegema, 1987). For the most part, however, decisions about the development of strategies and sequencing of activities had to be based on "best guesses" about what should be done. This often entailed the translation of local strategies to national actions and involved much invention.

In Figure 1 local strategies associated with each of the four organizing principles are presented. Following these local strategies abstracted from the literature is a description of the national level actions actually employed in the Families as Allies project.

Identify existing leadership and interest among individuals and organizations; begin to build a sense of community and a shared identity

At the local level, Staples (1987) describes talking with key "community gate keepers" to identify individuals who are leaders and who can provide access to other potential participants. Suggestions by Rothman and Reed (1984) about locating potential leaders and participants for community action regarding alcohol and drug problems include approaching parents and administrators through the public schools, clergy through local churches, and others through a variety of existing community organizations and structures. In local communities, one can often obtain lists of organizations through various directories, including the telephone yellow pages.

Ways of building a sense of community and a shared identity among local community members rely heavily on meetings (Rothman & Reed, 1984; Jay, 1984) and on techniques such as consciousness raising (Biklen, 1983). In 1984 there was no list of state and local parent organizations that included parents whose children had serious emotional problems, so one of the first project activities was to conduct a national telephone survey to locate and describe existing parent self-help and advocacy organizations throughout the United States. An important product of that survey was a national directory of local and state organizations that listed the services available, the geographic area served, information about newsletters, fees, and so on. One purpose of publishing the directory was so that leaders within parent organizations could learn about and find each other; isolation was clearly a problem, especially among fledgling groups. Another function of the directory was to provide a means by which individual parents in a given community could locate parent groups and each other.

In addition to publishing the national parent organization directory, other strategies to increase networking and to create a sense of community among parents included creation of an extensive data base and mailing list, and dissemination of regular bulletins and newsletters. In 1988-89 the Families as Allies project provided small grants to partially support five statewide parent organizations (four of which did not exist before the grants were available), and provided financial support, technical assistance, and evaluation to three more statewide parent organizations in 1989-90. This project also includes mechanisms for the leaders of these organizations to meet together and to communicate regularly.

Help community members obtain the necessary information and skills to engage in problem analysis, planning, and action

This step involves gathering information than can be used to promote needed change. In local communities the focus can either be on the locality, or neighborhood itself (Warren & Warren, 1977; Rubin & Rubin, 1986), or on the nature and extent of a specific social problem (Warheit, Bell & Schwab, 1977; Women's Crisis Center, Ann Arbor, 1979).

Activities undertaken by the Families as Allies project included a national survey of parents designed to gather information about their needs and their experiences with obtaining services (Friesen, 1989b), development of a parent handbook that includes information about parents' rights under current policies (Kelker, 1988), and training packages designed to help parents become more effective advocates (Kelker, 1987). Technical assistance about starting and maintaining parent groups and organizations is also provided by the Families as Allies project, as well as by others (Donner & Fine, 1987).

State and community level need assessments conducted by the various state CASSP projects and the development of a model comprehensive system of care (Stroul & Friedman, 1986) were also very important factors in providing necessary information to par-

FIGURE 1. Local and National Organizing Strategies Related to Project Organizing Principles

ORGANIZING PRINCIPLES	LOCAL STRATEGIES
IDENTIFY EXISTING LEADERSHIP AND INTEREST AMONG INDIVIDUALS; BUILD A SENSE OF COMMUNITY AND SHARED IDENTITY	Talk with key "community gatekeepers" to identify individual leaders who can provide access to other potential participants (Staples, 1987)
	Approach members through schools, churches & other community organizations (Rothman & Reed, 1984)
	Hold meetings to build a sense of community and shared identity (Jay, 1984), employ consciousness-raising techniques (Biklen, 1983)
HELP COMMUNITY MEMBERS OBTAIN NECESSARY INFORMATION AND SKILLS TO ENGAGE IN PROBLEM ANALYSIS, PLANNING AND ACTION	Gather information re: locality or neighborhood needed to promote change (Warren & Warren, 1977; Rubin & Rubin, 1986)
	Gather information about nature & extent of specific social problem (Warheit, Bell & Schwab, 1977)
	Provide training re: problem analysis & advocacy
ASSIST COMMUNITY MEMBERS TO IDENTIFY COMMON PURPOSES, GOALS AND ACTION PLANS	Hold community meetings, membership surveys, public hearings
HELP COMMUNITY MEMBERS CREATE AN ONGOING STRUCTURE WITHIN WHICH TO CONTINUE ORGANIZING AND ADVOCACY EFFORTS	Develop ways to meet members' needs, run effective meetings (Haggstrom, 1987; Kahn, 1982; Rubin & Rubin, 1986); attend to administrative aspects of running an organization (Kruzich & Austin, 1984)
	Coalesce local organizations to form national organizations (Hatfield, 1981; Roos, 1970)

ents. Attendance at national meetings by parents was also sponsored by some state CASSP projects, which gave parents from various parts of the country the opportunity to interact. During 1987 the National Mental Health Association and the National Alliance for the Mentally Ill also focused on children's issues for the first time in conjunction with their annual membership meetings.

ORGANIZING PRINCIPLES	NATIONAL STRATEGIES
IDENTIFY EXISTING LEADERSHIP AND INTEREST AMONG INDIVIDUALS; BUILD A SENSE OF COMMUNITY AND SHARED IDENTITY	Conduct a national telephone survey to locate and describe existing parent self-help and advocacy organizations
	Publish national directory of parent organizations to reduce isolation; parents can find parent groups and each other
	Create national mailing list; disseminate regular bulletins and newsletters
HELP COMMUNITY MEMBERS OBTAIN NECESSARY INFORMATION AND SKILLS TO ENGAGE IN PROBLEM ANALYSIS, PLANNING AND ACTION	Conduct national survey to learn about parents' needs and experiences; disseminate findings
	Develop parent handbook, training to help parents become effective advocates
	Provide technical assistance re: starting and maintaining parent support groups
ASSIST COMMUNITY MEMBERS TO IDENTIFY COMMON PURPOSES, GOALS AND ACTION PLANS	Sponsor regional and state conferences to develop action plans for improving services
	Hold national-level planning meetings to identify common concerns, directions
HELP COMMUNITY MEMBERS CREATE AN ONGOING STRUCTURE WITHIN WHICH TO CONTINUE ORGANIZING AND ADVOCACY EFFORTS	Promote development of local and statewide parent organizations
	Sponsor a national conference to form national network
	Give support to ongoing organizing efforts

Assist community members to identify common purposes, goals and action plans

Community meetings, membership surveys, and public hearings are common ways that local organizers use to accomplish this step. A primary mechanism employed at the national level was a series of regional and state conferences attended by delegations of parents, professionals, and in some instances, policy-makers. These meetings follow a common format and involve conference delegates in identifying goals, strategies for overcoming barriers, and action plans to be carried out post-conference (McManus & Friesen, 1986a). In many instances, these meetings stimulated the establishment of new parent groups and/or action efforts involving parents, professionals and other interested citizens. The Families as Allies project also held a meeting of parent leaders from across the U.S. to develop a set of recommendations for use by the U.S. Departments of Education (DOE), and Health and Human Services (HHS) in setting future directions and funding priorities.

Help community members create an ongoing structure within which to continue organizing and advocacy efforts

Organization-building is a frequently addressed topic in the community organization literature (e.g., Haggstrom, 1987; Kahn, 1982; Rubin & Rubin, 1986). This literature addresses locating members, meeting their needs and concerns, running effective meetings, as well as the administrative aspects of maintaining a community organization (Kruzich & Austin, 1984). Little information about how to stimulate the formation of a national organization is available. Lessons about how other national organizations formed often describe "bottom up" approaches that involved the coalescing of local existing organizations (e.g., Hatfield, 1981; Roos, 1970). Because few local organizations existed, the strategy employed by the Families as Allies project, in concert with state CASSP programs, was to promote the development of local parent groups while working toward the establishment of a national network.

In December, 1988, sixty parents and professionals from twenty states met together to consider "next steps" in the organizing process, with an explicit goal of at least laying the groundwork for a national network. At that meeting, parents from around the country voted to form a steering committee to consider what form a "national voice for children" should take. Some favored a separate, new organization, others preferred to link with one or more existing organizations, while others wanted a coalition of existing national, state, and local organizations. Although there was considerable disagreement over the form that an "organized national voice" should take, there was widespread agreement among parents and professionals that such a voice is sorely needed, and impressive energy available to work toward that goal. Subsequently a majority of the members of the steering committee voted to form a new national organization and the Federation of Families for Children's Mental Health was legally incorporated in August, 1989.

Ensuing chapters in this history must await future developments. With the formation of the steering committee and the birth of a new organization, however, the Families as Allies project completed at least the first phase of this organizing effort (Blum & Ragab, 1985).

STIMULATING LARGE-SCALE CHANGE

This change effort involving the organization of parents whose children have serious emotional disorders suggests that large scale (state, regional, national) organizing can be accomplished, given a situation in which there is a felt need for change and a shared change goal. The example described in this article also had other favorable conditions—a federal initiative on behalf of childrens' mental health, a national and state structure promoted through the CASSP grants, and eventually, resources with which to conduct necessary research, communicate widely with prospective participants, and bring parents together periodically. This change effort should not, however, be viewed as idiosyncratic, and material resources were not the most important ingredient.

The most fundamental requirement was the belief that national change was possible. The process of creating large-scale change aspirations was necessary for Families as Allies staff, for parents, and for the community of professionals who wanted to see services for children and families improved. For Families as Allies staff, the process of "aspiration-raising" was accelerated by having contact with leaders in parent and professional organizations that have a national focus including self-help and advocacy groups, and by a familiarity with the literature on social change, social movements, community organization, social planning, and social administration.

Although there is some indication that social workers of today are less likely to have social action goals than was the case in the 1960's (Reeser & Epstein, 1987), there are other indications that human service professionals are increasingly recognizing the importance of advocacy and empowerment for themselves as well as their clients (Hegar & Hunzeker, 1988; Pinderhughes, 1983; Wintersteen & Young, 1988).

It may also be important to re-examine the assumption held by many community organizers that "true" change can only be brought about by those who have a clear and unwavering commitment to a conflict model of practice (see, for example, Galper and Mondros, 1980). As discussed earlier, this change effort, although rooted in a social action (or conflict) philosophy, employed a wide mixture of strategies, many of which could be most accurately described as consensual and cooperative. Models that blend the best aspects of community organization, self-help and consumerism may hold promise for promoting important changes in service delivery quality and capacity, although they admittedly stop short of restructuring the basic distribution of resources in our society. Ongoing vigilance against cooptation and goal displacement is, of course, necessary when working "within the system" (Lamb, Hoffman, Hoffman & Oliphant, 1986). This is an ongoing concern for the new, resource-poor Federation of Families for Children's Mental Health that becomes especially salient when decisions about from whom to seek and accept funds must be made.

Propositions for thinking about large-scale change. The following propositions may be useful to practitioners, administrators, and other students of change when thinking about "aspiration-raising" and when preparing for other steps in the change process:

1. Opportunities exist, or can be created, to promote large scale change efforts.
2. Promotion of large scale change aspirations and acquisition of requisite knowledge and skills should be a part of the competencies of all social work practitioners. Thus, they should be a part of the social work educational experience for all students, but should be particularly emphasized for those specializing in macro practice.

3. Social and intellectual isolation of social workers and social work students exacerbates a tendency to "think small."
4. Change aspirations are more likely to be limited to those that are small and/or local when social workers and students lack information about or experience with large scale change efforts.
5. The process of creating large-scale change aspirations, developing a knowledge base and skills for large scale change for social work practitioners, faculty, and students involves a process of empowerment.

Given these propositions, a number of different strategies might be developed to promote change aspirations, and to locate or develop necessary change strategies and techniques. Experience with a state or national change effort is key to developing the belief that such change is possible, and that the social worker can contribute to and influence the change effort. Therefore, practitioners, students and faculty members are encouraged to get involved in an ongoing large-scale change process. If direct involvement is not feasible, the student of change can develop a plan for staying informed about developments in a field or interest area (e.g., get on mailing lists, keep abreast of the pertinent literature, choose to focus academic assignments or research projects in the area).

Those who aspire to engage in large scale change efforts will undoubtedly be able to think of many other possibilities for learning about and promoting state and national level change. For practitioners, students, and faculty, alike, involvement in such efforts can be an exciting and empowering experience.

REFERENCES

Bersani, H. Advocacy: The role for parents' groups. *The Exceptional Parent*, 1985, *15*, 28-30.

Biklen, D.P. *Community organizing: Theory and practice.* Englewood Cliffs, NJ: Prentice-Hall, Inc., 1983.

Blum, A. & Ragab, I. Developmental stages of neighborhood organizations. *Social Policy*, 1985, *15*(4), 21-28.

Caplan, P.J. & Hall-McCorquodale, I. Mother-blaming in major clinical journals. *American Journal of Orthopsychiatry*, 1985, *55*(3), 345-353.

Donner, R. & Fine, G. *A guide for developing self-help/advocacy groups for parents of children with serious emotional problems.* Washington, DC: Georgetown University Child Development Center, Child and Adolescent Service System Program, 1987.

Dunst, C.J. & Trivette, C.M. Enabling and empowering families: Conceptual and intervention issues. *School Psychology Review*, 1987, *16*(4), 443-456.

Friesen, B.J. (Ed.). *Working with families of the mentally ill: A handbook.* Salem, OR: Oregon Mental Health Division, 1984.

Friesen, B.J., Griesbach, J., Jacobs, J.H., Katz-Leavy, J. & Olson, D. Improving services for families. *Children Today*, 1988, *17*(4), 18-22.

Friesen, B.J. Parents as advocates for children and adolescents with serious emotional handicaps: Issues and directions. In R.M. Friedman, A.J. Duchnowski & E.E. Henderson (Eds.), *Advocacy on Behalf of Children with Serious Emotional Problems.* Springfield, IL: Charles C Thomas, 1989a.

Friesen, B.J. *Survey of parents whose children have serious emotional disorders: Report of a national study.* Unpublished research report, Research and Training Center on Family Support and Children's Mental Health, Portland State University, 1989b.

Friesen, B.J. & Koroloff, N.M. Family-centered services: Implications for mental health administration and research. *The Journal of Mental Health Administration*, 1990, *17*(1), 13-25.

Galper, J. & Mondros, J. Community organization in social work in the 1980's: Fact or fiction? *Journal of Education for Social Work*, 1980, *16*(1), 41-48.

Haggstrom, W. The tactics of organization building. In F.M. Cox, J.L. Erlich, J. Rothman, & J. E. Tropman (Eds.), *Strategies of community organization*, (4th ed.). Itasca, IL: Peacock, 1987.

Hatfield, A. The organized consumer movement: A new force in service delivery. *Community Support Service Journal*, 1981, *2*, 3-7.

Hegar, R.L. & Hunzeker, J.M. Moving toward empowerment-based practice in public child welfare. *Social Work*, 1988, *33*(6), 499-502.

Jay, A. How to run a meeting. In F.M. Cox, J.L. Erlich, J. Rothman & J.E. Tropman (Eds.), *Tactics and techniques of community practice*, (2nd ed.). Itasca, IL: Peacock, 1984.

Kahn, S. *Organizing: A guide for grassroots leaders.* New York: McGraw-Hill, 1982.

Kelker, K. *Taking charge: A handbook for parents whose children have emotional handicaps* (2nd ed.). Portland, OR: Research and Training Center on Family Support and Children's Mental Health, Portland State University, 1988.

Kelker, K. *Making the system work: An advocacy workshop for parents.* Portland, OR: Research and Training Center on Family Support and Children's Mental Health, Portland State University, 1987.

Klandermans, B. & Oegema. D. Potentials, networks, motivations, and barriers: Steps towards participation in social movements. *American Sociological Review*, 1987, *52*, 519-531.

Klieman, M.A., Mantell, J.E. & Alexander, E.S. Collaboration and its discontents: The perils of partnership. *The Journal of Applied Behavioral Science,* 1976, *12*(3), 403-410.

Knitzer, J. *Unclaimed children.* Washington, DC: Children's Defense Fund, 1982.

Kruzich, J.M. & Austin, M.J. Supervision and management in community organization agencies. In F.M. Cox, J.L. Erlich, J. Rothman & J.E. Tropman (Eds.), *Tactics and techniques of community practice* (2nd ed.). Itasca, IL: Peacock, 1984.

Lamb, H.R., Hoffman, A., Hoffman, F. & Oliphant, E. Families of schizophrenics: A movement in jeopardy. *Hospital and Community Psychiatry,* 1986, *37*(4), 353-357.

Lindblom, C.E. The science of muddling through. In N. Gilbert & H. Specht (Eds.), *Planning for social welfare: Issues, models, tasks.* Englewood Cliffs, NJ: Prentice-Hall, Inc., 1977.

Lloyd, I. Don't define the problem. *Public Administration Review,* 1978, *38,* 283-286.

Lourie, I. Presentation to Child and Adolescent Service System Program (CASSP) directors, Washington, DC, March 12, 1990.

McManus, M. & Friesen, B. (Eds.), *Families as allies: Conference proceedings.* Portland, OR: Research & Training Center on Family Support and Children's Mental Health, Portland State University, 1986a.

McManus, M. & Friesen, B. (Eds.), *Parents of emotionally handicapped children: Needs, resources, and relationships with professionals.* Portland, OR: Research and Training Center on Family Support and Children's Mental Health, Portland State University, 1986b.

Modrcin, M. Emotionally handicapped youth in transition: Issues and principles for program development. *Community Mental Health Journal,* 1989, *25*(3), 219-227.

National Advisory Mental Health Council. *A national plan for research on child and adolescent mental disorders.* Washington, DC: National Institute of Mental Health, 1990.

Olson, D. A developmental approach to family support: A conceptual framework. *Focal Point,* 1988, *2*(3), 3-6.

Pinderhughes, E.G. Empowerment for our clients and for ourselves. *Social Casework,* 1983, *64*(6), 331-338.

Reeser, L.C. & Epstein, I. Social workers' attitudes toward poverty and social action: 1968-1984. *Social Service Review,* 1987, *6*(4), 610-622.

Roos, P. Parent organizations. In J. Wortir (Ed.), *Mental retardation: An annual review,* Vol. 2. Orlando, FL: Grune & Stratton, 1970.

Rothman, J. Three models of community organization practice, their mixing and phasing. In F.M. Cox, J.L. Erlich, J. Rothman & J.E. Tropman (Eds.), *Strategies of community organization* (3rd ed.). Itasca, IL: Peacock, 1979.

Rothman, J. & Reed, B.G. Organizing community action to address alcohol and drug problems. In F.M. Cox, J.L. Erlich, J. Rothman & J.E. Tropman (Eds.),

Tactics and techniques of community practice (2nd ed.). Itasca, IL: Peacock, 1984.

Rubin, H.J. & Rubin, I. *Community organizing and development.* Columbus, OH: Merrill, 1986.

Saxe, L., Cross, T. & Silverman, N. Children's mental health: The gap between what we know and what we do. *American Psychologist*, 1988, *43*(10), 800-807.

Silver, S., Friedman, R.M., Duchnowski, A.J. & Kutash, K. *Findings from the national adolescent and child treatment study of seriously emotionally disturbed children: Implications for assessment and delivery of care.* Unpublished research report. Tampa, Florida: Research & Training Center for Children's Mental Health, University of South Florida, 1988.

Smith, M.J. & Moses, B. Social welfare agencies and social reform movements: The case of the single parent family. *Journal of Sociology and Social Welfare*, 1980, *7*(1), 125-136.

Staples, L. "Can't ya hear me knocking?": An organizing model. In F.M. Cox, J.L. Erlich, J. Rothman & J. E. Tropman (Eds.), *Strategies of community organization* (4th ed.). Itasca, IL: Peacock, 1987.

Stroul, B. & Friedman, R. *A system of care for severely emotionally disturbed children and youth.* Washington, DC: CASSP Technical Assistance Center, Georgetown University Child Development Center, 1986.

Warheit, G.J., Bell, R.A. & Schwab, J.J. *Needs assessment approaches: Concepts and methods.* Washington, DC: Government Printing Office, 1977.

Warren, R.B. & Warren, D.I. *The neighborhood organizer's handbook.* Notre Dame, IN: University of Notre Dame Press, 1977.

Wintersteen, R.T. & Young, L. Effective professional collaboration with family support groups. *Psychosocial Rehabilitation Journal*, 1988, *12*(1), 19-31.

Women's Crisis Center, Ann Arbor. Organizing a Women's Crisis Center. In F.M. Cox, J.L. Erlich, J. Rothman & J.E. Tropman (Eds.), *Strategies of community organization* (3rd ed.). Itasca, IL: Peacock, 1979.

Young, T.M. Therapeutic case advocacy: a model for interagency collaboration in serving emotionally disturbed children and their families. *American Journal of Orthopsychiatry*, 1990, *60*(1), 118-124.

Rebuilding the Human Services:
The Profession Mobilizes
for Social Work in Public Education

Rose Starr, DSW
Robert Schachter, DSW

In the fall of 1985 the social work community in New York City faced the threat of declassification of social work positions in the special education division of the public school system. A major commission report not only assailed the need for professional social work expertise in required special education assessments, but it also criticized the lack of attention to preventive services for the general school population (Commission on Special Education, 1985). As a result, the New York City Board of Education implemented a plan to reduce the number of social workers in special education, assign major social work assessment and case management functions to special education teachers, and divide the responsibilities of the remaining social workers between general and special education students.

The New York City Chapter of the National Association of Social Workers, with a small staff, attempts to maintain a large array of membership-initiated committees. However, routine handling of

Dr. Starr is Associate Professor, Hunter College School of Social Work, The City University of New York, 129 East 79th Street, New York, NY 10021. Dr. Schachter is Executive Director of the New York City Chapter of the National Association of Social Workers.

An earlier version of this paper was presented at the Association on Community Organization and Social Administration Symposium, Annual Program Meeting, Council on Social Work Education, Chicago, 1989.

the social work crisis in special education was insufficient to reverse the Board of Education challenge. New initiatives were required to establish priorities for Chapter activities and engage Chapter board of directors and members in a comprehensive mobilization of resources within and beyond the profession.

This article reports on the design and results of the professional association's action strategies to: (1) reverse the immediate threat to social workers' positions in the school system, and (2) establish permanent professional positions and functions in the public education system.

THE NATIONAL CONTEXT

With the publication of the report of the National Commission on Excellence in Education and its now famous alert that the nation is "at risk," the average citizen is aware of the failure of public education to prepare all students to enter the world of work and to perform the basic activities of citizenship (National Commission on Excellence, 1983). The negative implications for the country's ability to compete in the world economy have received broad media and public policy attention.

Social workers take pride in having a long term association with both the field of education and the functioning of local school systems. School social work has been a specialization since 1906 (Costin, 1987). In the late 1980s, 12,000 professionals identified themselves as school social workers and practiced in public school settings throughout the nation (NASW Commission on Education, 1987). They have responded to the challenge of the Commission on Excellence at a national level by establishing an Education Commission at NASW, and devoting increased resources and attention to the issue. Locally, school social workers have participated with school and community-based professionals in addressing such problems as truancy, dropping out, child abuse and neglect, and crime, as well as challenges associated with ethnic and cultural diversity, new immigrant populations and English as a second language (Gonet, 1990; Schwartz, 1988; Wodarski & Hedrick, 1987; Allen-Meares, Washington & Welsh, 1986; Famiglietti, Fraser & Newland,

1984; Waltzer, 1984; Harris, 1983; Winters & Easton, 1983; Colca, Lord & Colca, 1981; Jirsa, 1981; Bellos, 1974).

While these efforts reflect a firm commitment of the profession, historically and currently, to the field of education, it is also true that on federal and local levels, the relationship of social work to public education is tenuous. As recently as 1982 the Reagan administration sought to delete social work services from the regulatory definition of related services in P.L. 94-142, the Education for All Handicapped Children Act. According to Freeman (1982), social work services were vulnerable because they were clearly defined in regulations, but not in statute. Similarly, Title I of the federal Education, Consolidation and Improvement Act (1965), providing educational assistance to low income children, permits but does not mandate social work intervention in the education of poor children. It is left to local school districts to choose to allocate scarce educational resource dollars across multiple instructional and non-instructional functions.

In such a competitive arena, optional social work services are not only vulnerable, but often may not be considered for inclusion. In recent years, in response to fiscal constraints or the personnel choices such restraints require; school districts in New Orleans, Colorado, Arizona, and Rochester as well as New York City, have threatened or carried out cuts in school social work positions. If social work services are poorly understood or underdeveloped, they are likely to suffer disproportionately in this process (Levine, 1984).

SOCIAL ACTION FOR SCHOOL SOCIAL WORK

Through the National Association of Social Workers and independent state associations of school social workers, the profession has engaged in a variety of activities to advance the role and status of school social work personnel and services. Nationally and locally, these organizations have fought cuts in P.L. 94-142 and Title I of the Education Consolidation and Improvement Act. They have lobbied to maintain social work services and providers as components in both statute and regulation (Freeman, 1982; Hare, 1988; McCullough, 1985). Collaboration with the National Alliance of

Pupil Services Organizations has been a conscious strategy in these efforts (Freeman, 1982; Hare, 1988).

However, the range of social action activities of NASW chapters has been relatively limited. The focus tends to be on the development and dissemination of social policy statements, legislative lobbying and provision of testimony. Furthermore, intervention has been targeted primarily at the national level. There have been few organized efforts by social workers to participate in local government hearings and board of education meetings, or to influence education policy makers and elected officials. Similarly, the media rarely have been used to focus public attention on social work concerns in the field of education (McCullough, 1985).

The dominance of licensure and vendorship as continuing association priorities since the mid-1970s has appeared to constrain more comprehensive pursuit of other goals and the resources needed to achieve them, including those related to school social work (Lause, 1979; Saxton, 1988).

EDUCATION POLICY
AND LOCAL POLITICAL INFLUENCE

According to Barbaro (1980), the advancement of school social work requires the development of social workers into a politically influential interest group at the local level. Viewing educational decision-making as highly political, pluralistic and competitive, Barbaro emphasizes the importance for social workers to shape educational decisions affecting school social work services in local school districts through development of political knowledge, skills, and alliance building.

Using Easton and Massialas, Barbaro presents a systems framework for understanding educational decision-making at the local level. In his opinion, social workers do not always recognize the potential for decision-making influence as one of the multiple actors presenting demands or resources which must be responded to by such key decision-makers as the commissioners of education, local boards of education and school system superintendents. Thus, they are rarely a consistent part of the political process generating specific policy decisions. Second, they often fail to recognize that educational commissioners at the state level and superintendents at the local level hold considerable formal and discretionary power over the direction educational programs take.

Although Barbaro uses these insights to suggest a variety of political influence-building activities for individual social workers, the components and dynamics of the framework he defines can also be applied to the activities of professional organizations. It is from this conceptual base that we now turn to an analysis of the mobilization of social workers by the New York City Chapter of NASW to rebuild a professional service structure in the New York City public schools.

SOCIAL WORK DECLASSIFICATION IN THE NEW YORK CITY SCHOOL SYSTEM

There was a substantial social work presence in the New York City school system through an institutionalized clinical service program, Bureau of Child Guidance (BCG). Employing hundreds of MSWs, psychologists and psychiatrists, BCG was dismantled in 1978 due to the cumulative effects of at least four factors: the City's fiscal crisis, the implementation of P.L. 94-142 providing clinical and support services to children requiring special education, the growing dissatisfaction of educators with the orientation and results of this inhouse clinical service, and the growing interest of community organizations in providing mental health services to school children and their families.

Subsequently, social workers were employed through the special education system to provide social assessments of referred children and to function as the case manager of the multi-disciplinary assessment team. Few social workers were available to the general school population and, even in special education, the prescribed functions did not conform to generally-accepted definitions of professional practice.

With the publication in 1985 of "A Call For Quality" by the New York City Mayoral Commission on Special Education, reform of the system was demanded as documentation was presented of the inappropriate placement of children (largely minorities) in "dead end," stigmatized education programs. Key recommendations focused on developing preventive services in general education and reorienting special education to narrower educational versus clinical goals.

Following the Mayoral Commission's logic (and required by a longstanding settlement from a judicial decree to comply with federal and state regulations on timely and appropriate placement of children referred for special education services), the New York City Board of Education implemented a plan to restructure the multidisciplinary team, termed the "Enhanced Model." The restructuring removed social workers as formal members of the team, retaining them half-time in special education for the purpose of initial social assessments only. The remainder of their time was to be spent in general education providing preventive services. In this way, the Board planned to both increase the overall number of two-person assessment teams and cut down on the flow of referrals to special education. However, attrition of 35-40% of the existing social work workforce of 483 was an integral part of the Board's model, thus undermining the effectiveness of the plan. As a result, the assessment teams were comprised of only school psychologists and teachers designated to perform academic assessments, titled educational evaluators. The latter were assigned case management and on-going social assessment responsibilities previously carried out by social workers.

PROFESSIONAL MOBILIZATION: STRATEGY DEVELOPMENT

In the face of these dramatic changes, school social workers were relatively isolated individually and collectively as a professional discipline. There was great hope that the teacher's union (in which the social workers formed a small professional chapter together with school psychologists) would represent their cause at higher levels. As a result, any concerted effort by school social workers at the grassroots level to influence the emerging declassification scheme was limited in nature and scope prior to the Board's formal announcement and, to some extent, was focused on encouraging the union to respond.

At the NASW Chapter level, actions were taken that conformed with generally-accepted patterns of response to threatened standards or constituents. Meetings were held; position statements and letters were conveyed to key Board personnel, politicians and advocates. These standard political pressure tactics (Rubin & Rubin, 1986), however, fell far short of what objectively was required to halt an exceedingly strong Board of Education initiative that had both philosophical and institutional support. With the formal announcement of the new "Enhanced Model" and Chapter recognition that school social work staff cutbacks and a diminished professional role were imminent, new strategies were necessary.

In order to address the threat to social work in the public schools, four interrelated strategies were consciously planned to position NASW to influence the decision-making process (Tropman & Erlich, 1979). The *intraorganizational* strategy aimed to build consensus within the Chapter about the need to take action and to determine how to make resources available for action to occur. The second, the *definitional* strategy, was a corollary of the first. Redefining issues and shaping perceptions was fundamental to achieving consensus among the leaders of the organization (Staples, 1984). It was also necessary for achieving consensus among school social workers and other members of the profession as well as gaining support from the decision makers in the education arena (Staples, 1984). This last group of actors, the decision makers, were ultimately the targets of the third and fourth strategies aimed at the *judiciary* and *political* systems where the authority for setting policies resides (Staples, 1984). All four strategies were interactive.

While these judicial and political strategies can be characterized as, respectively, defensive and offensive, both were dependent for their development upon the foundation provided by the first two. Thus the Chapter's strategic planning highlights the "means-ends" chain in goal achievement, in which strategies meant to realize particular objectives are themselves instruments in successive phases of the organization's conscious change efforts (Tropman & Erlich, 1979). The development of Chapter cohesion and consensus through the intraorganizational strategy was a planned means toward the achievement of judicial or political goals.

The primary mode of influence integral to all four Chapter strategies was inducement rather than force or agreement (Tropman &

Erlich, 1979; Staples, 1984). Through its presentation of expertise and issues as well as the garnering of increased constituent and political support, the Chapter hoped to improve its ability to persuade key decision makers to listen to and act on its claims. Thus, Chapter strategies can be seen as part of an overall planning process (Staples, 1984) in which successive levels of influence-building were geared to "getting an issue on the policy agenda" (Rubin & Rubin, 1986) and gaining increased recognition as a necessary and useful party in the development of solutions.

INTRAORGANIZATIONAL STRATEGIES

Underpinning the development of a more substantial and focused organizational initiative was the growing consensus of Chapter leadership about the need to be more effective in policy arenas directly affecting social work practice. Increasingly, dissatisfaction was expressed with the Chapter's limited involvement in numerous issues without discriminating levels of importance or assessing possible impact. The Chapter's reactive stance, often committing resources "too little and too late," was also subject to criticism.

A principle emerged that paved the way for new organizational strategies to address environmental challenges to the profession, including the school social work crisis: the Chapter should anticipate and act on public policy trends and decisions that directly affect social work practitioners and their clients. As a corollary, the Chapter's role is critical when other organizations can not be relied upon to take action in the profession's behalf. It was expected that Chapter membership would respond enthusiastically to initiatives that reflected this principle.

This expectation was borne out by the rapid mobilization of both the Chapter Board of Directors and the school social work constituency. The solid support of the Board of Directors was obtained. The challenge to school social workers was viewed as a Chapter priority to which substantial resources for defense should be committed.

Given the Board of Director's active support, the reactivation of a small School Social Work Committee was both possible and necessary. Guided by the principles of self-help and self-determination, NASW as a membership organization expected that school social workers (as those most directly affected) would spearhead the fight and raise money necessary to carry it forward. As a result, a network of school social workers was established encompassing the majority of school districts in New York City. A new active leadership core took responsibility for expanding the network, communicating the need to take unified action, and identifying the practice consequences of the Board of Education's plan. It also undertook a fund raising drive through which approximately $10,000 was raised from individual school social workers themselves.

The reorganization of Chapter priorities, including the mobilization of a specific membership constituency, in response to a threat to the profession had never before been attempted by the Chapter. Thus, these intraorganizational strategies represented the onset of a new direction, more streamlined and assertive than what preceded.

REDEFINING THE ISSUES

One of the impediments to social workers organizing in their own behalf in the face of Board of Education cutbacks and job restructuring was the perceived lack of credibility of their cause. Little value was placed on the availability of social workers in the school system. This was due to a lack of understanding of the contribution social workers make to education, a perception that social workers were not adequately deployed and the availability of social workers in community-based organizations. As a result, many in the education and social service communities interpreted efforts to resist the Board's actions as simply self-serving efforts to save jobs, rather than a response to a social need. While attempting to save jobs was viewed as legitimate by social workers as union members, some considered it questionable for a professional association. In short, a body of conventional wisdom had emerged that supported reform of the system in particular directions. In this context, social worker activity was viewed as resistance to positive change or maintenance of an untenable *status quo*.

These attitudes created an environment in which the ethical basis for professional organizing was questioned. As a result, social workers themselves were not unified on the rightness of their position, and the organizing effort began with extreme obstacles to overcome, both within and beyond the professional community.

To address this situation additional strategies to redefine the problem and to articulate the profession's position were formulated (Rubin & Rubin, 1986; Staples, 1984). First, Chapter leadership systematically identified and presented the educational implications of social, cultural and familial factors absent from the Board of Education's purview. The case was made for the inseparability of education and the social environment.

Specifically, the Chapter articulated the crucial role of the social worker in providing culturally-relevant, psycho-social assessments for the multi-disciplinary evaluation team. Given the racial, cultural and linguistic bias known to affect the special education assessment process, the costs to the family and child of inappropriate assessment, diagnosis and placement were highlighted. The involvement of parents and the maintenance of due process rights in the special education determination process were also emphasized.

In a second component of the strategy, we distinguished the quality of services provided by the special education system from their quantity. The court, the Board of Education and some educational advocacy groups, although in disagreement on many issues, were unified in assigning priority to the improvement of the productivity of the special education system. Thus, from their perspective the design of procedures and systems to eliminate the long-standing backlog in assessments of children referred for special education services was paramount. Their emphasis was limited to increasing the number of personnel assigned to assessment teams, rather than the qualifications needed for a comprehensive team approach. To counter this, the Chapter argued that more efficient processing of students was meaningless if the substantive nature of the contact failed to result in a full, fair and culturally-relevant understanding of the child in his/her milieu. In short, the rationale for social workers on the team was based on their contribution to a quality process and result. Without this, a rather flat, one-dimensional picture of the child could be expected at best; at worst, the child's future could be jeopardized by inadequate or biased judgments.

A third part of the strategy was geared to members of the profession rather than the broader education community. In this component, the school social work crisis was defined as professional declassification in which all social workers — not just those working in schools — have a vested interest. Specifically, the features of the school social workers' struggle were presented as generalizable and common to other major fields of practice, rather than unique and limited to school social workers alone. This formulation of the problem was an essential ingredient in the effort to unify a profession, frequently focussed on its differences.

Shaping perceptions of the issue in these ways made it possible to unite the profession and mobilize its resources. This strategy also recast the nature of the problem in the special education system and thus provided the basis for the Chapter's judicial arguments opposing the Board of Education's proposals. Perhaps most importantly, focusing on quality and cultural-relevance enabled the Chapter to counter the accusation of self-interest as the primary motivation for action. Given the politics of social services in education, however, the Chapter continues to confront the suspicion that its efforts serve the profession alone, rather than the public interest.

JUDICIAL STRATEGY

The intraorganizational and definitional strategies discussed above laid the foundation for redress of social worker declassification through the courts. Although the Board of Education exercised control over the special education program, the policy and personnel shifts inherent in the Board's Enhanced Model required approval by Federal district court. The salience of this influence led to a decision by the Chapter to insert itself into the ongoing judicial process affecting special education.

Begun in 1979 with the *José P.* class action suit, the court issued a judgment against the New York City Board of Education for failing to comply with Federal and State law and regulations requiring education for all handicapped students. The *José P. vs. Ambach* class action suit was brought on behalf of all handicapped children living in New York City, aged 5-21, who had not been promptly evaluated and placed in appropriate programs by the New York City Board of Education. Specifically, the Board was directed to provide adequate and timely assessments of children referred for special education services and to establish an interdisciplinary team and due process procedures for this purpose. Failure to comply brought the Board back to court on many occasions. At the point the Enhanced Model was introduced to eliminate the backlog in assessments, the backlog was 29,000 cases.

Investigation of the history and mid-1980s status of José P. made it clear that the Chapter could present its case to the court through the mechanism of an *amicus curiae* brief (Schlozman & Tierney, 1986). To pursue this strategy the Chapter decided to hire a lawyer in the Fall of 1986 and to underwrite the legal costs, with the understanding that membership fundraising would ultimately cover these expenditures. In letters to the Court seeking *amicus* status, the Chapter stated its concerns about the Enhanced Model and presented the need for a quality assessment process, knowing that the primary parties in the case were focusing exclusively on quantitative issues (i.e., the elimination of the backlog in cases through increases in productivity, workload or personnel). Thus the intent was to both provide information and advocate a point of view (Schlozman & Tierney, p. 372).

In January 1987, the Federal judge issued a decision granting the Chapter *amicus* status and ordered a hearing on two questions: (1) whether removal of the social worker from key roles in the assessment team would have a deleterious effect on the assessment process, and (2) whether social workers should be hired to fill team positions in the likely event that insufficient numbers of psychologists and educational evaluators were available. He further ordered an end to the attrition of social workers already initiated by the Board of Education.

The opportunity for a judicial hearing provided the profession a welcome platform for a presentation on the contribution of social workers to quality client service. Three social workers representing direct service, supervision and social work education provided evidence and were cross-examined by Board of Education lawyers. An educational evaluator testifying for the United Federation of Teachers supported the NASW position.

In April 1987, the Judge ordered the immediate hiring of ninety social workers for service solely in special education. On the other hand, he refused to overturn the Enhanced Model, granting the

Board of Education as the executors of the special education program more time to demonstrate its projections for the Model. Nevertheless he acknowledged the "substantial and disturbing" testimony provided by NASW, ordered the Board of Education to provide additional evidence on the viability of its projections for reducing the backlog, and stated that, based on the evidence thus far, the Enhanced Model might be incapable of improvement. He further suggested that the Board consider quality of service issues in its future planning.

During the 1987-88 school year, a second hearing was convened strictly on the adequacy of the Board's ability to reduce the backlog of cases. As a result of growing skepticism with the Board's plan, the magistrate recommended that the Enhanced Model be overturned and that the multi-disciplinary team including the social worker, be restored. Specifically he advised an increase in the numbers of assessment team professionals, including 100 more social workers.

At this point, the Board of Education entered out-of court negotiations with the José P. plaintiffs to settle the case prior to a final order by the Judge. The resulting agreement increased the numbers of educational evaluators and psychologists so that an evaluation team would be available in every school.

From the beginning the Chapter viewed the judicial strategy with hopefulness as the first positive option available. At the same time, this initiative thrust the profession into unfamiliar and turbulent waters in which there was risk of a negative decision and little certainty as to the advantage the process would ultimately provide (Rubin & Rubin, 1986). Although court action did not achieve a reversal of the Board of Education's position on the future utilization of social workers in special education, judicial activity halted the Board of Education juggernaut and prevented a knockout blow to school social workers. More importantly, it acknowledged the legitimacy of quality of service issues and announced the arrival of a new if modest actor on the special education scene. With a relatively small investment, in fact this strategy yielded major outcomes in jobs saved or added (Schlozman & Tierney, 1986).

POLITICAL STRATEGY

As the court process unfolded, it became clear that the judiciary and its powers exist in, shape and are shaped by a political context (Rubin & Rubin, 1986). Thus, the court was loathe to overstep its bounds and take aggressive action toward the educational designates of a duly elected City executive unless and until it was perfectly clear that such designates were totally incapable of meeting their public mandate. The court was also sensitive to an emerging consensus on what might be workable or could reasonably be required of the Board of Education and — by extension — the City in added costs as well as external authority. The Board of Education and José P. plaintiffs were equally attuned to the avoidance of extreme positions that would anger the court and invite an unwanted decision.

The out-of-court settlement by the primary parties emerging from these dynamics proved pivotal for the Chapter. Not only did it confirm the limitations of NASW participation in the judicial process, it further illuminated the importance of the broader political context and the extent to which social work was not a factor in education policy in New York City. In fact, the profession had neither the credibility nor the resources to significantly influence long-term decisions in the education arena. Court action on which we had laid our hopes and been fortunate beyond expectation could be preempted in the "real world."

This painful realization led to the development of a political strategy that continues today and coincided with the expansion of the Chapter's concern for the needs of children school-wide as well as in special education. The goal was to improve and expand the utilization of social work services in the public school. To achieve this goal, the Chapter embarked on three interrelated processes: (1) fact-finding and program design on state-of-the art social work and support service models in public schools; (2) outreach to educational and other influentials to build a constituency for social work in public education; and (3) fund-raising to expand NASW staff resources devoted to advocacy in education.

To raise money, Chapter staff and leaders pursued private funding sources. A proposal to the United Way in New York City resulted in a grant to hire a consultant to further program and constituency development activities. To gain support for an enhanced professional role in public education, the Chapter initiated discussions within the social work community and beyond. The New York State Association of Deans of Social Work Schools and the Legal Defense Fund of NASW responded with significant contributions and organizational assistance. Accordingly, an advisory committee was organized to expand the Chapter's base of participation and support from social work educators, executives of child and family service agencies, and politicians with close ties to the profession.

Initial efforts to persuade actors in the education community of the efficacy of social work services yielded crucial information on the attitudes and perspectives within that sector. Specifically, meetings with Board of Education officials (most notably the President and a former Chancellor), education advocates, and the United Federation of Teachers helped clarify the status of social work and the priorities of the educational system. Key influentials and decision-makers emphasized the need to enhance educational achievement system-wide, to prevent over-reliance on a flawed special education system, and to rebuild "guidance" service decimated during the City's fiscal crisis. We learned, furthermore, that several factors impeded rational planning to improve utilization of mental health professionals, including social workers, in the schools: a multiplicity of funding streams, the lack of coordinating structures within the system and between school and community, and the inadequacy of resources overall. While individual social workers were often lauded, as a discipline social work was not viewed as a priority. There was, however, growing concern that the City's children receive a better education and that, to this end, an expanded and effective social support network be devised.

Recognizing these views and priorities, the Chapter broadened its perspective. It reshaped its goals to advocate for a comprehensive social support system designed to meet the unique needs of local school districts and implemented to better utilize an array of existing resources in both school and community. Offering itself as a catalyst toward system-wide planning and problem-solving, the Chapter has continued to seek foundation funding to gain support for this approach and to identify the elements of workable service models.

In this regard, proposal writing has yielded foundation grants underwriting modest additional staffing to coordinate constituency-building efforts. Chapter leaders have met with key Board of Education personnel (including now-deceased Chancellor Richard Green), political, legislative and parent leaders, resulting in invitations for Chapter participation on Board of Education committees and programs. New relationships with local districts and schools have been forged, resulting in requests for technical assistance collaboration and consultation.

FROM DEFENSIVE TO OFFENSIVE STRATEGIES: AN ANALYSIS OF COSTS AND BENEFITS

What began as an effort to defend the role and position of social workers in special education evolved into a proactive agenda by the New York City Chapter of NASW to develop a viable environment for social work practice and the social needs of children in the school system as a whole.

As the New York City experience highlights, different problems, potentials, and prerequisites are associated with defensive and offensive efforts.

This case study corroborates the experience of community activists who find that stopping an unwanted action may be easier to achieve than instituting an innovative change or plan. Although a positive outcome was not predetermined at the outset, the Chapter defense of school social workers can be considered modestly successful. Clearly, the social work role in the special education assessment process has been diminished. However, the Chapter was able to hold the line on overall numbers and through a court order, gain an injection of 80 new workers into the system.

Several elements appear responsible for this outcome. First, the stakes for the profession were high, and, as a result of Chapter work on issue definition, were understood as such. The Board of Education's new plan was portrayed as an all-out assault on social work in special education that left the profession only two alternatives: fight the assault or accept the end of a social work role and presence in this area of practice. Chapter members came to recognize that remaining aloof or passive in the face of this degree of external threat would have forcefully confirmed the vulnerability of the profession to the decisions and interests of others.

Declassification of social work positions or their preemption by workers with differing education and orientation, furthermore, would have serious results not only for social work personnel but also for the quality of service provided a low-income, culturally diverse, problem-plagued population. The spectre of these dire consequences, together with the absence of other advocates within or outside the social service and education communities, impelled the Chapter to act. These same factors enabled the Chapter to galvanize its members, garner resources and pursue a plan and strategies for defense.

Additional factors facilitating the Chapter's defense were the availability of internal resources, the specificity of the target for change, and the preexisting lawsuit against the Board of Education. Long-standing federal court involvement in the New York City special education system provided a ready-made vehicle for change and an environment of criticism of Board actions on which the Chapter could build. Although several of the powerful plaintiffs in the case did not support Chapter objectives, the information in their complaint assisted the Chapter in its own (Rubin & Rubin, 1986). Furthermore, in the development of witnesses and testimony, the United Federation of Teachers became an important public ally whose support school social workers, as union members, could claim.

The financial resources obtained from member donations, National NASW and State Dean's Association grants, and others, generally kept pace with the legal fees necessary to participate in the lawsuit (Rubin & Rubin, 1986). The Chapter brought other resources to bear as well, most notably its members' expertise in providing court testimony, making the case for the social work role, and redefining the issues for allies and opponents alike.

With the court case as the primary vehicle for defense, the target of change was clear and singular. Chapter advocacy was focused on changing Board of Education decisions as outlined in its revised plan for the operation of special education services (Staples, 1984).

The court as intermediary in this change was the primary factor enabling Chapter efforts to achieve some level of success. As we have seen, although the judiciary is not immune to the preferences of key actors, it can take an independent stand based on objective data and its interpretation of the law.

If the court case and related judicial strategy were the engines of the Chapter's defense, the political strategy was the primary means for pursuing its pro-active agenda. Through this agenda, the Chapter recognized and sought to change the inadequate representation of the profession within the Board of Education establishment from central to district and school levels. It understood that the special education conflict was the tip of the iceberg: social workers and the social work profession were perceived as marginal contributors to the educational enterprise and thus vulnerable to cutbacks or de-classification system wide.

In the New York City example, the factors promoting success of the Chapter's defensive activities limited its accomplishments in the offensive arena. Goals and targets for change were less clear and specific. Galvanizing the Chapter to support long-term, complex and open-ended influence-building efforts was more difficult. The intellectual arguments in behalf of a comprehensive social support system were considerably less compelling than the emotional plea to save jobs and services.

Subgroups within the Chapter with different interests and perceptions questioned the direction of the effort and the resources necessary to achieve it. Some leaders opposed the shift in focus toward advocacy for a comprehensive multi-disciplinary service system, preferring a singular emphasis on gaining more respect and positions for social workers alone. Others were concerned about whether increased resources for support services in the schools would provide jobs for Board of Education-employed (school-based) social workers or social workers from community-based organizations on contract with the schools. Still others did not view education advocacy as a chapter priority with claims on Chapter resources equivalent to such mainstream social work practice areas as health or child welfare.

The absence of sustained unity had implications for the level of resources that were available. Although some Chapter staff time was allocated, the thrust was towards financing project personnel through outside grants. This meant that the education advocacy consultant, once hired, spent as much time on maintenance efforts seeking funds as pursuing project goals. The follow-through and continuity necessary to nourish evolving relationships in the education policy arena were contingent on the success of parallel fund raising efforts.

Since their inception, the Chapter's offensive efforts remain embryonic in development. To play a more active role requires long-term involvement in education policy and the politics of social service provision at the local level. As the New York City experience suggests, however, an activist stance directed toward system change is extremely difficult to implement. The culture of many NASW Chapters may not support this kind of activity, given its costliness in time, staffing and money, and the press of other perceived priorities. As well, in an era of constraint and competition, social work advocates in education do not enter a level playing field and may not be able to surmount the advantage and claims of those actors already "at the table."

The political process responds to numbers, money and influence. Thus, the dilemma: effectiveness in the political arena may have more long term pay off for social work, but may be harder to achieve, given the profession's mission, lack of money, influence and numbers relative to others competing in the same field of interest.

FUTURE DIRECTIONS

To enable the Chapter to be more effective in the future, the factors limiting support, resources and unity will need to be addressed. Certainly the Chapter would benefit from engaging outside allies (Rubin & Rubin, 1986). In a highly contested area like education, a *coalition* strategy, built on current political efforts, may be the only route for a professional association like NASW to gain acceptance of its argument. In the New York City case, there are four likely allies: the union representing all pupil personnel disciplines in the school system, the associations representing diverse professionals and administrators, consumer or advocacy organizations representing the school system's parents and students, and community social service agencies with interests in school-based services. If this strategy is pursued, ongoing assessment of means and ends will be required to identify what NASW may have to offer in exchange for such coalition support and what may be compromised as a result.

Furthermore, the enduring tension between a professional association as a "self-interest" trade association and an "advocate for children and quality service" will need to be sensitively handled for collaboration and coalition with others to occur. "Trade association" sponsorship of advocacy efforts may hurt their political acceptability and the redefinition of issues. In turn, the lack of political clout limits an association's ability to gain acceptance of its perspectives. Alignment with others perceived as less "self-interested" — in an arena characterized by interest group politics — may be one solution to this dilemma as long as the policies and programs pursued do not stray too far from the profession's central concerns.

With respect to resources, professional social workers have been inadequately socialized to the relationship of sizeable dues and association membership to advocacy for professional issues and mission. There is a need to teach students while in social work school that their goals are contingent on effectiveness in the political process. Only with greater numbers and financial resources will the profession's association, NASW, be in a position to exercise increased independent influence with respect to its message and definition of issues. Social workers must be more prepared to "put their money where their values are" if they wish to achieve this result.

Although many factors may deter social workers from joining their professional association, one may be the suspicion that its interests may not be consonant with the client good. The debate on who benefits from licensure (the restriction of service), for example, has helped fuel this concern. Empirical data are needed on the connection between issues affecting the profession (e.g., declassification, low salaries) and their impact on clients. Such information may help clarify when interests are dissonant or consonant and perhaps narrow the gap perceived between advocacy for clients and one's self as a professional.

The field must also address the disunity within the social work profession, based on its diversity in auspices and fields of practice, and the oppositional organizational interests these create. Social work students and practitioners should become aware of the policy issues and politics they will confront, often with negative impact on professional unity. In the public education arena discussed in this article, the organizational competition between public-employed school-based social workers and those from voluntary, community-based organizations must be understood and addressed in a constructive way. Leadership and education are needed to develop an appropriate professional position in the client's interest.

REFERENCES

Allen Meares, P., Washington, R.O. & Welsh, B.L. *Social work services in schools.* Englewood Cliffs, NJ: Prentice-Hall, Inc., 1986.

Barbaro, F. School social work: the politics of professional survival. *Social Work in Education*, 1980, *3*, 5-17.

Bellos, N. *Innovative projects in school social work practice.* Syracuse, New York: Syracuse University, 1974.

Colca, L.A., Lord, S.A. & Colca, C. Responding to the challenge of school integration. *Social Work in Education*, 1981, *4*, 40-49.

Commission on Special Education. *Special education: A call for quality.* New York: Office of the Mayor, 1985.

Costin, L. School social work. *Encyclopedia of Social Work*, 18th edition, 1987, 532-545.

Famiglietti, J.F., Fraser, M.W. & Newland, K.E. Delinquency prevention: Four developmentally oriented strategies. *Social Work in Education*, 1984, *6*, 259-273.

Freeman, M. Reaganomics and school social work. *Social Work in Education*, 1982, *4*, 69-71.

Gonet, M. A three-pronged approach to substance abuse prevention in a school system. *Social Work in Education*, 1990, *12*, 208-216.

Hare, I. School social work and its social environment. *Social Work in Education*, 1988, *10*, 218-234.

Harris, L.H. Role of trauma in the lives of high school dropouts. *Social Work in Education*, 1983, *5*, 77-88.

Jirsa, J.E. Planning a child abuse referral system. *Social Work in Education*, 1981, *3*, 7-22.

Lause, T. Professional social work associations and legislative action. *Journal of Sociology and Social Welfare*, 1979, *6*, 265-273.

Levine, R.S. Barriers to the implementation of P.L. 94-142. *Social Work in Education*, 1984, *7*, 22-34.

McCullough, J.G. School social work issues: an analysis of professional association actions. *Social Work in Education*, 1985, *7*, 192-203.

NASW Commission on Education. *School social workers: Serving children at risk*. Silver Spring, MD: National Association of Social Workers, 1987.

National Commission on Excellence in Education. *Nation at risk: The imperative for educational reform*. Washington, DC: U.S. Department of Education, 1983.

Rubin, H.J. & Rubin, I., *Community organizing and development*. Columbus, OH: Merritt Publishing Company, 1986.

Saxton, P.M. Vendorship for social work: observations on the maturation of the profession. *Social Work*, 1988, *33*, 197-201.

Schlozman, K.L. & Tierney, J.T. *Organized interests and American democracy*. New York: Harper and Row publishers, 1986.

Schwartz, S. School-based strategies for the primary prevention of drug abuse. *Social Work in Education*, 1988, *11*, 53-63.

Staples, L. *Roots to power: A manual for grassroots organizing*. New York: Praeger Publishers, 1984.

Tropman, J.E. & Erlich, J.H. Strategies: Introduction. In F.M. Cox, J.L. Erlich, J. Rothman & J.E. Tropman (Eds.). *Strategies of community organization: A book of readings* (3rd ed.). Itasca, IL: F.E. Peacock publishers, 1979.

Waltzer, F. Using a behavioral group approach with chronic truants. *Social Work in Education*, 1984, *6*, 193-200.

Winters, W.G. & Easton, F. *The practice of social work in schools*. New York: The Free Press, 1983.

Wodarski, J.S. & Hedrick, M. Violent children: a practice paradigm. *Social Work in Education*, 1987, *10*, 28-42.

Mental Health Reform:
A Case Study of Influencing
Social Policy
Through Legislation and Litigation

Stephen P. Wernet, PhD

INTRODUCTION

Major revisions of the Texas Mental Health Code were enacted in 1983 by the State Legislature. These changes resulted from the work of a Task Force commissioned in 1981 by the Texas Legislature. The charge to the Task Force was to review and recommend revisions of the Texas Mental Health Code. The Code which had been enacted in 1958 had become antiquated due to: (1) the advances in and routinization of medication in treating mental illness; (2) the shift from institutional care to community-based care of the mentally ill; and (3) the expansion of the legal rights of the mentally ill (Mental Health Code Task Force Report, 1983).

The work of the Mental Health Code Task Force (hereafter called the Task Force) produced two pieces of legislation. These were the Texas Mental Health Code and the Orders of Protective Custody (OPC). These were known, respectively, as Senate Bill 435 (SB 435) and Senate Bill 213 (SB 213).

OPC was one of the major changes in the 1983 revisions of the Texas Mental Health Code although it is only one component of it.

Dr. Wernet is Assistant Professor, School of Social Work, University of Illinois at Urbana-Champaign, Urbana, IL 61801.

The author acknowledges the support provided for the research by Kathryn Moss, PhD and the Hogg Foundation for Mental Health.

OPC outline the hearing procedures for probable cause. These are the procedures through which an individual is involuntarily committed into a mental health facility for observation.

The OPC section of the Mental Health Code was originally enacted on February 23, 1983 as emergency legislation Senate Bill 213 (SB 213). It was passed in response to a class action lawsuit which challenged the due process procedures for involuntary commitments. This case is known as *Luna v. Van Zandt*. The remarkable fact concerning SB 213 is that it was conceptualized, drafted, revised, submitted, heard, and passed by both houses of the Texas Legislature in 32 days!

Many previous attempts to revise the Mental Health Code had failed in either the Legislature or in coalitional meetings. The swift passage of SB 213 demonstrated that this rare political feat could be achieved in a legislative session. What is especially remarkable, however, was the simultaneous passage of a second piece of legislation (SB 435), the Mental Health Code revisions. These two legislative successes can be attributed to the work of the same coalition, the Mental Health Code Task Force.

This article outlines the process of influencing and changing social policy. The research was concerned with the nature of the interaction between the Task Force, the courts, the legislature, the public agencies, and other special interest groups. The research attempted to identify the key actors involved in the legislative process, to outline the flow of events surrounding the passage of SB 213, to outline the rewards and costs for advocates and opponents of SB 213 and to identify the resources which were aggregated on behalf of the passage of SB 213.

THEORETICAL BACKGROUND

The development of social policy and the passage of legislation are political processes. Numerous attempts to explain the collective behavior of political processes have been espoused over the past decade. Utmost, however, social policy and the passage of legislation are interpersonal processes that depend upon meaning and negotiation that seek change in the social structure elements. There are several theories through which one can understand and analyze these processes. These theories include resource mobilization, social exchange and negotiation theories. They discuss similar phenomena but with slightly different emphases. When combined, these theories yield three concepts for analyzing the influence process and explaining change.

First, there are the *structural contexts*, i.e., the larger transcending or historical circumstances that bear upon a coalition (Strauss, 1982; Maines, 1979). Structural contexts encompass the social, political and economic environments within which a coalition is founded as well as their impact throughout the history of the coalition. This includes the general organizational history or roots of the organization, how it grew and the pattern of exchange relationships (Roberts-DeGennaro, 1987). It has been shown that a direct relationship exists between pre-existing organization or solidarity and success of political change efforts (Gamson, 1975; Barkan, 1979; Jenkins & Perrow, 1977; Fireman & Gamson, 1979).

Second, *negotiation contexts* are the relevant features of the immediate setting (Maines, 1982; Strauss, 1982). This is the interorganizational realm. There are four components to this context. The first is the *role of the coalition* in the community. The second component is the *resource condition* of the coalition. It includes such items as political power, support, and manpower as well as the more traditional, fiscal resources. Research has shown that improved resource conditions is a key factor in increased and successful political activity (Jenkins & Perrow, 1977; Jenkins, 1977; Barkan, 1979; Lipsky, 1968). One of the necessary resources is someone who is willing to invest time and effort in the hope of a preferred outcome (Zald & McCarthy, 1975; McCarthy & Zald, 1977; Fireman & Gamson, 1979; Sink & Stowers, 1989). The third component of the negotiation context is the *policy window* (Sink & Stowers, 1989). This is defined as an opportune period of time during which change can be achieved for a given social issue. The final component of the negotiation context is the *triggering mechanism* (Sink & Stowers, 1989). This is known as an event(s) which helps to create an environment favorable to policy change. This event(s) may be general, enduring over time and repetitive, or specific, solitary and intense.

The third and final factor is *negotiation processes*, the actual types of interaction engaged in by participants (Maines, 1979; Strauss, 1982; Zurcher, 1983). This is the intraorganizational or interpersonal arena within a coalition. These are the observable characteristics of the coalition, i.e., the formal and informal, personal styles of the participants. This includes the interpersonal relationships and interactions which exist both between and among the members of the negotiation process. The standard patterns for resolving basic and recurring problems and conflicts, i.e., the bargaining process, within and without the coalition, is of particular interest in this factor (Thompson, 1967; Lipsky, 1968; Zald, 1969; McLanahan, 1980; Mathiasen, 1983).

The collective behavior of social policy development can be understood through analysis of the influence process. The explanation of change should focus upon three elements: the structural contexts, the negotiation contexts, and the actual negotiation processes. The structural contexts describe the historical stage upon which a contemporary change effort will rest. The negotiation contexts describe the immediate, contemporary background within which a change effort will be attempted. The negotiation processes describe the interpersonal interactions within which the problem-solving work takes place.

METHODOLOGY

A snowball sampling technique was implemented for identifying both key informants and pertinent documents. Several waves of individuals involved in the Task Force were asked to identify the key actors instrumental in the effort to draft and pass SB 213. Seven individuals were identified as key informants and interviewed. The interviewees included a state hospital superintendent, a staff person for the SB 213 sponsor, the Chair of the Task Force, the opposing attorneys in the class action suit, *Luna v. Van Zandt*, and two Probate Court judges.

Numerous documents were analyzed during the research. These

included four drafts of SB 213, the draft of SB 435, the Attorney General's file concerning the class action suit, internal Texas Department of Mental Health and Mental Retardation (TDMHMR) memoranda concerning the class action suit and numerous memoranda from the Task Force concerning SB 435 and SB 213.

For semi-structured interviews, a standardized introduction and a core set of questions were asked of all interviewees. The core questions focused upon the following issues: (1) the quick passage of emergency legislation, (2) the Task Force's concern with the probable cause procedure prior to the lawsuit being settled, (3) the advantages and disadvantages of SB 213, (4) the judges' refusal to issue Orders of Protective Custody, (5) the wording of the law, and (6) the keys actors involved in facilitating the passage of SB 213. The judges, the Chair of the Task Force, and the opposing attorneys in the class action suit were posed additional questions seeking (1) clarification about specific events and facts concerning the class action suit, and (2) the chronology of events and processes among the key actors.

The data from both the interviews and documents were aggregated, coded and analyzed through the use of analytic description (Lofland, 1985). Comparisons were made among various versions of the legislative bills and the then-existing law.

FINDINGS

The chronology of events which encompass the enactment of SB 213 are a compact scenario which has historical antecedents dating to 1979. Figure 1 depicts these interrelationships.

Structural, Historical Contexts

Predating the 1983 legislation, there were several attempts to revise the Texas Mental Health Code. These started in 1978 and ended in the defeat of a code revision in the 1979 Legislative session. This defeat was attributed to various aspects of the revision being objectionable to a variety of people.

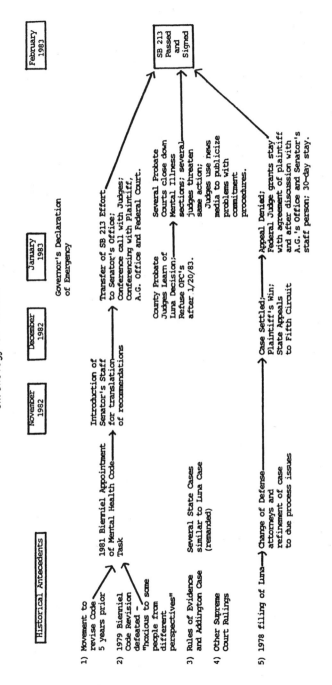

Figure 1
Chronology of Events

The Lawsuit

Also, in 1978, the lawsuit, *Luna v. Van Zandt,* was filed in the Texas State Courts. This lawsuit was filed during an era of class action suits. Like many other cases of this era, *Luna v. Van Zandt* sought to protect and guarantee the civil rights of individuals from a disadvantaged class, i.e., the mentally ill. The environment was conducive to protecting individual rights as well as revising legal codes in favor of greater individual protection.

Because of staff turnover, the plaintiff's attorney, a public defender, changed during the lawsuit. The new public defender chose to focus the class action suit along the issues of due process. That is, the class action lawsuit sought to indemnify the plaintiff, Luna and the eligible class, for arbitrary and unreasonable incarceration in a mental health facility. According to various sources, this issue refinement helped to focus the class action lawsuit and facilitate the legal process.

Mental Health Code Task Force

Prior to the 1981 sitting of the Legislature, a public interest attorney had coalesced a group of advocates, service providers and ex-patients who sought revision of the Mental Health Code. This group pursued and achieved the appointment of an interim study group, i.e., the Mental Health Code Task Force, by the Legislature in 1981. The purpose of the Task Force was to enhance the constitutionality and efficiency of the due process procedures within the Mental Health Code as well as increase programs for locally-based outpatient care. The Task Force worked on revising and updating the Mental Health Code from June 1981 through November 1982.

Thirty-five different groups were represented within the Task Force. These various special interests dichotomized into two major practice conflicts: rights of clients versus need for treatment, and community-based services versus institutional-based care. A logjam developed because of the conflict between these advocate interests. The polarization centered around the Orders of Protective Custody that are the procedures through which people enter the mental health system. On one side, there was concern for protecting the individual and his/her choice for community treatment, while the other side advocated protecting the community and removing individuals to total care facilities. For either group to compromise too readily would have resulted in loss of prestige and influence.

The Task Force subdivided into various working committees concerned with revising various sections of the Mental Health Code. Although no official delegates represented the various groups, several spokespersons emerged and were described as natural leaders. In particular, five key actors were identified: a Legislative aide, the Chairperson of the Task Force, a legal scholar, the public interest attorney, and a State Hospital Superintendent. The first three actors were perceived as fair and understanding both sides of the logjam; the other two actors were seen as representing, respectively, clients' rights and need for treatment.

Court Decisions

Concurrent to the Task Force's work, there were several Supreme Court and Appellate Court rulings which established legal precedent. The Supreme Court cases addressed rules of evidence, as well as guarantee of both equal protection and the right of due process. Several cases which addressed these same issues were pending at various levels of Texas State Courts. In fact, it was stated that on several occasions hearings on the *Luna v. Van Zandt* class action suit were postponed at both attorneys' request in order to wait for lower courts' rulings. However, none of the outstanding court cases and/or appeals resulted in settlement of the due process issue represented by *Luna v. Van Zandt*.

The structural/historical context surrounding the passage of SB 213 was rich and ripe. There were parallel processes occurring simultaneously in the legal and legislative arenas between 1978 and 1983. The legal environment was an active, adversarial one focusing upon civil rights of disenfranchised groups, including the mentally ill. Out of several unsuccessful legislative efforts came an action-set (Roberts-DeGennaro, 1987) which successfully negotiated the Task Force appointment in 1981. The action-set structure was broadly representative and inclusive. This seems to have resulted in a sense of mutual understanding and communication among the various interest groups. The pattern of exchange relationships consisted of delegated responsibility and working committees over a 17-month period. The action-set, however, appears to have splintered into two opposing groups, rights versus treatment advocates, which centered upon the crux of the Task Force's work, orders of protective custody.

Negotiation Contexts

The Task Force had reached a critical junction in November 1982. The coalition that comprised the Task Force had unraveled. It seemed to have reached an impasse. At this point, however, two incidents occurred that reinvigorated the Task Force's work. First, the effort to draft emergency legislation, i.e., the Orders of Protective Custody (SB 213), was transferred from one legislator to the Senator who was also the primary sponsor of the Mental Health Code revision (SB 435). The consolidation of the mental health legislation sponsorship provided unified and coordinated leadership on behalf of these initiatives. Second, the Senator who was sponsoring SB 435 (and now assumed sponsorship for SB 213) assigned one of his aides as staff person to the Task Force. The aide's function was to facilitate the translation of the Task Force's findings into legislation. This aide was dually trained as a community psychologist and a lawyer. This enabled him to converse with both sides of the conflict, i.e., legal or rights advocates as well as provision or service advocates. The aide, in collaboration with four members of the Task Force, drafted the initial revision of the Mental Health Code (SB 435) in December 1982.

Also, in December 1982, *Luna v. Van Zandt* was settled in Federal Court in favor of the plaintiffs, i.e., Luna. After a denial of the State's appeal to the Fifth Circuit Court, the Court Order was scheduled to go into effect on January 26, 1983. If the Court Order had gone into effect, the TDMHMR would have been without any procedures for involuntary commitments to its institutions.

At the end of December 1982, the Probate Court Judges, who have jurisdiction in mental health law, learned of the Luna decision. They initiated discussions among themselves. These continued throughout January 1983. They also attempted, unsuccessfully, to discuss the case with the Federal Court in order to gain some opinion concerning their role for proper implementation of the ruling. The Justices' discussion among themselves focused upon their personal liability in committing people to state hospitals without due process. Several justices refused to make mental health commitments. This effectively disrupted the mental health commitment process in their jurisdictions. Several other justices threatened such action. Several justices contacted the news media concerning the absence of Orders of Protective Custody procedures for committing mentally ill persons to state hospitals.

The negotiation context surrounding the passage of SB 213 was rich and ripe. The role of the Task Force in the political community was well established. Its composition was considered representative of the various and interested constituents. It was defined as the legitimate mechanism for legislative action concerning mental health issues. Two events further enhanced the resources within the negotiation context. The consolidation of legislative sponsorship increased the political resources. The assignment of a staff aide who assumed task leadership increased the personnel resources. The policy window was provided by the settling of the class action suit, *Luna v. Van Zandt*. The triggering mechanism for negotiations was the disruption of mental health commitments by the Probate Courts' justices. In conjunction with the subsequent and quick denial of the State's appeal, these two events constrained the various interest groups and forced them to coalesce sooner than if a prolonged appeal had occurred.

Negotiation Processes: Key Actors of the Action Set

The eight key actors can be separated into two groups: those who were directly involved in SB 213 and those who were involved in the Mental Health Code revision (SB 435). (See Figure 2.) There were four individuals who were coterminous with the Task Force, the SB 435 effort and the SB 213 effort—the legislative aide, the Chair of the Task Force, the Assistant Attorney General and the public interest lawyer. The other four individuals were involved exclusively with a single issue, a constitutional lawyer served on

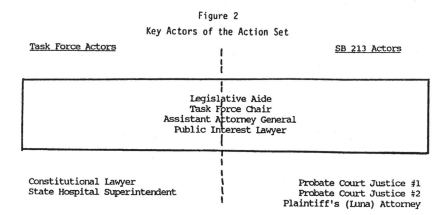

Figure 2
Key Actors of the Action Set

the Task Force, while two urban Probate Court justices and the plaintiff's attorney were concerned with SB 213.

The legislative aide's role is clear. Because of his professional training as both a community psychologist and a lawyer, the legislative aide was able to span the key constituencies of client advocates, service providers and jurists. It was his work that served to facilitate the negotiation process. His work "behind the scenes" served to move the processes along. He translated the Task Force's recommendations into legislative form; he initiated conference calls with the Probate Court justices; his longstanding friendship with the plaintiff's attorney seems to have facilitated the agreement for a court stay; he negotiated the professional organizations' support for SB 213.

The other three coterminous actors were prime examples of the power to influence a social system. The Chair of the Task Force brought "intelligence, sophistication and credibility"; the constitutional lawyer brought "twenty-five years of jurist perspective and practice as well as intellectual abilities to synthesize"; the public interest lawyer brought credibility as the "organizer of a coalition of advocates and providers."

Three of the single issue actors brought incentive threats and external impetus to the negotiations. The plaintiff's attorney brought the authority of the Federal judiciary. The two Probate Court justices brought the power to impact directly the gatekeeping mechanism of the mental health system. The Probate Court justices were a keystone in breaking the standoff. Their uncertainty and anxiety concerning malpractice and liability was quite high. It was their potential losses or costs which resulted in the coalesced support of SB 213 and its ultimate passage.

As the deadline approached, it was these eight individuals who served as the architects for a final piece of legislation. Individually, each actor represented a major constituency or perspective. Collectively, they represented the sum of constituencies concerned with the issues at hand. The coalescing occurred because every constituency was willing to compromise in order to reach a solution. The work was completed because the actors were the most interested, available, thoroughly knowledgeable and trusted people involved in the process.

The dynamics of the negotiating process of this work group seem to have been a major advantage for confronting and diffusing the conflicting interests which could have subverted the Task Force's work. With deadlines nearing and work incomplete, the group employed an informal arrangement for accomplishing its task. Conference calls were held by the judges and the Senator's Office concerning drafts of SB 213; similar tactics were employed with the plaintiff's attorney, the Attorney General's office and the Federal Court. As a result of these latter conference calls, a thirty day stay was granted by the Federal Court with agreement of the plaintiff's attorney. The Governor declared a state of emergency, thereby bypassing numerous procedural protocols and allowing this proposed legislation to be immediately heard.

SB 213 was heard, reported out of committee and passed on the floors of both houses of the Texas Legislature in late January and early February. On February 23, 1983, the Governor signed SB 213 into law—three days short of the Federal Court's stay deadline.

The successful negotiations were dynamic and contingent upon several items. A core group emerged within the action set. It consisted of key actors who were seen as legitimate representatives of the various constituencies in the action set. The core group was coterminous with two different but related work efforts (SB 213 and SB 435). There was a single agent, the legislative aide, who served as a key facilitator of the work of this core group. He was credible to all interest groups. He was perceived and functioned as an invested but disinterested party to the work. There were incentive threats and external impetus simultaneously prodding the negotiations.

DISCUSSION OF FINDINGS

As one interviewee stated, "It's just that it ended up being a compromise." This seems to be the highest compliment that could be attributed to the entire process. The codification effort had a structural, historical context that was largely unsuccessful. The actors who coalesced around the work of the Mental Health Code revision became involved because of the principles or interests which they sought to codify. What resulted in 1983 was a solution that was acceptable to all members of the coalition.

The negotiation context was an unusual configuration of elements that came together in a timely, albeit unexpected, fashion. Unlike past legislative efforts, one of the principal differences in this successful outcome was the improved resources within the negotiation context. The resource enhancement included intangible resources, e.g., political support, political favors, opportunity, and professional reputations, as well as tangible resources, e.g., money, staff personnel, and court action deadlines.

The first resource improvement was greater costs or incentive threats. The cost for the protagonists was the Mental Health Code; the cost for the antagonists was professional reputation. For these antagonists to derail SB 213, it would have entailed blocking an emergency declaration by the Governor and risking loss of valuable resources such as political favors and money. These costs, however, were also opportunity conditions that effected the negotiation process. Both protagonists and antagonists alike could advocate for their respective viewpoints while conceding some ground because of their knowledge of the other parties' constraints.

The second resource improvement was greater political power. The influence of the Senator and the prestige of the Task Force Chair were vital to the work. Because of the group composition, the Task Force had an established credibility with outside observers and interest groups.

The third resource improvement was the concurrent general and specific policy windows that developed into an opportune time for change. The trigger mechanism which was also a policy window was both specific and compelling. This observation corroborates Sink and Stowers' (1989) finding concerning the triggering mechanism. It appears likely that a specific, compelling policy window is a necessary condition for successful policy outcomes. These enhancements produced both time and awareness in the service of the legislative efforts. Time "allowed things to blend together into this proposal" (Chairperson, 1983; Legislative Aide, 1983). The trigger mechanism, which was an external constraint, produced an awareness "that some change was inevitable and stonewalling was no good" (Superintendent, 1983; Legislative Aide, 1983).

The fourth resource improvement was dedicated personnel. The legislative aide was someone who understood all of the issues and, therefore, could span all interest groups. His facilitative behavior was instrumental in building coalitions, resolving conflicts and achieving consensus.

Finally, the establishment of an action-set (Roberts-DeGennaro, 1987) that consisted of all the known, important players was crucial to the eventual success of the legislative activity. Communication, understanding and mutual trust were catalyzed through the internal dialogue of the Task Force. These prolonged, interpersonal interactions facilitated the negotiations' processes. A sense of trust evolved among the group that each member was working to include everyone's concerns. These prolonged, interpersonal interactions also generated credibility between the work group, Task Force members and extra-Task Force parties. They were instrumental in the evolution of both a representative work group approach to the Task Force and an informal structure. A sense of trust was generated which allowed for the small work group to not only draft the recommendations of the Task Force but to also rapidly develop the draft of SB 213.

Unlike the findings of Sink and Stowers (1989), the structure and process of the exchange network was critical to its success. As one interviewee stated, "If it weren't for these personal relationships and prior exposure to significant others, then it is unlikely that SB 213 could have progressed as rapidly and as neatly as it did." The final version of SB 213 was acceptable to all parties because everyone believed that each member was working towards a maximization of every interest group's concerns in the final proposal.

IMPLICATIONS FOR SOCIAL WORK PRACTITIONERS

Several implications for social work practice can be culled from these findings. First, practitioners should acquire and maintain brokering and bargaining skills. The arenas of mediation and conflict resolution can provide the practitioner with ready experience and training for skill acquisition and refreshment. An integral part of these skills is the ability to fairly represent all sides of the issue to each party.

Second, practitioners should focus upon maintenance of forums which provide for ongoing interpersonal interaction between parties of disparate opinions on a given issue. This type of forum builds mechanisms of communication, facilitating both understanding and trust. When an opportunity presents itself, therefore, a mechanism for dialogue would be in place, thereby reducing the likelihood of loosing the opportunity to stimulate change or reduce tensions.

Third, investment of some resources are crucial for successful outcomes. At a minimum, the tangible resource of dedicated personnel must be infused into the work process. These personnel must have credibility with and acceptance from the various interest groups. Intangible resources of incentive threat and external sanction or credibility are also a necessary condition for success. External sanction or credibility indicates the public vesting of authority in the work group thereby creating a greater likelihood of acceptance for the outcomes. If all parties to the issue have something to lose, then all parties will have something to gain by a timely and successful outcome.

Finally, the practitioner needs to be vigilant for opportunities. They are usually time-limited. In particular, knowledge of the triggering mechanisms can often aid in identifying opportunities for change. It is also important for practitioners to become skilled in assessing external impetus for change. Through linking opportunity and external impetus, a practitioner may be able to stimulate change in a given situation.

CONCLUSIONS

Several conclusions and recommendations can be culled from this study. First, there must be substantial resource improvement in the negotiation context in order to catalyze social policy change. These improvements include dedicated personnel, political power, credibility and recognition, a compelling policy window plus real time barriers with associated incentive threats and opportunity costs for all parties. Second, there must be an action-set of actors who interact over a prolonged period of time.

For practitioners and educators interested in changing social policy and teaching the associated skills, several recommendations derive from the findings. It is sufficient for the successful practitioner to possess three sets of skills. Proficiency in the skills of identifying and assessing substantive issues and resources in the political environment are necessary. The second skill set focuses upon resource development. These include developing the aforementioned resources as well as development of interpersonal, communication forums for on-going dialogue among disparate interest groups. The final set of skills concern intervention and mediation of conflicts. Bargaining and brokering skills are necessary for the successful practitioner. Therefore, the competent social change agent will have substantive knowledge about the sufficient conditions for social change as well as possess sufficient skills for facilitating the change process.

REFERENCES

Barkan, S. Strategic, tactical and organizational dynamics of the protest movement against nuclear power. *Social Problems*, 1979, 27, 19-37.

Fireman, B. and Gamson, W. Utilitarian Logic in the Resource Mobilization Perspective. In M. Zald and J. McCarthy. (Eds). *The Dynamics of Social Movements: Resource Mobilization, Social Control and Tactics.* Winthrop Publishers, 1979.

Gamson, W. *The Strategy of Protest.* Homewood, IL: Dorsey Press, 1975.

Jenkins, J.C. What Is To Be Done: Movement or Organization? *Contemporary Sociology.* 1977, 8, 222-228.

Jenkins, J.C. & Perrow, C. Insurgency of the powerless: Farm workers movements (1946-1972). *American Sociological Review*, 1977, 42, 222-228.

Lipsky, M. Protest as a political resource. *American Political Science Review*, 1968, *62*, 1144-1158.

Lofland, J. and Lofland, L. *Analyzing Social Settings. Second Edition.* Belmont California: Wadsworth Publishing Company, 1985.

Maines, D. Mesostructure and social process. *Contemporary Sociology*, 1979, *8*, 524-527.

Maines, D. In search of mesostructure: Studies in the negotiated order. *Urban Life*, 1982, *11*, 267-279.

Mathiasen, K. *The board of directors is a problem: Exploring the concept of the following and leading boards.* Washington, DC: Management Assistance Group, 1983.

McCarthy, J. & Zald, M. Resource mobilization and social movements: A partial theory. *American Journal of Sociology*, 1977, *82*, 1211-1241.

McLanahan, S. Organizational issues in U.S. health policy implementation: Participation, discretion and accountability. *Journal of Applied Behavioral Sciences*, 1980, *16*, 354-369.

Mental Health Code Task Force. *Mental Health Code Task Force Report.* Unpublished Report, Austin, TX, 1983.

Roberts-DeGennaro, M. Patterns of exchange relationships in building a coalition. *Administration in Social Work*, 1987, *11*(1), 59-67.

Sink, D.W. & Stowers, G. Coalitions and their effect on the urban policy agenda. *Administration in Social Work*, 1989, *13*(2), 83-98.

Strauss, A. Interorganizational negotiation. *Urban Life*, 1982, *11*, 350-367.

Thompson, J. *Organizations in action.* New York: McGraw Hill, 1967.

Zald, M. The structure of society and social service integration. *Social Science Quarterly*, 1969, *50*, 557-567.

Zald, M. & McCarthy, J. Organizational intellectuals and the criticism of society. *Social Service Review*, 1975, *49*, 344-362.

Zurcher, L. *Social Roles.* Beverly Hills, CA.: Sage, 1983.

PART 4: ENHANCING EDUCATION IN COMMUNITY ORGANIZATION AND SOCIAL ADMINISTRATION

Strategies for Enhancing Administration Concentrations in Schools of Social Work

Barbara A. Pine, PhD
Lynne M. Healy, PhD
Myron E. Weiner, MGA

In recent years, there has been a decline in the number of graduate social work students selecting concentrations in administration. Moreover, fewer schools of social work now offer an administration major than in the past (CSWE, 1989). The resulting diminished pool of social workers who are professionally trained in manage-

Dr. Pine is Associate Professor, Dr. Healy is Associate Professor, and Mr. Weiner is Professor, School of Social Work, University of Connecticut, 1798 Asylum Avenue, West Hartford, CT 06117.

An earlier version of this paper was presented at the Association on Community Organization and Social Administration Symposium, Annual Program Meeting, Council on Social Work Education, Reno, 1990.

ment may mean that fewer human services agencies will be led by social workers in the future. Managers of these agencies will increasingly be trained through masters programs in business (MBA), public administration (MPA), non-profit management, or have no management training at all unless the social work profession launches an effective campaign to reverse these trends.

The underlying premise of this article, which suggests strategies for dealing with the above problems, is that the best preparation for managing a human service agency is graduate social work training in which the knowledge, values and ethics of the profession are integrated with the skills of modern management technology and leadership. The case for social work trained administrators has been eloquently stated elsewhere (Patti, 1984; Teicher, 1985). This article explores factors associated with the declining numbers of social work administration programs and of applicants to the remaining programs. A series of strategies undertaken by faculty in one school of social work is presented as an example. These strategies were designed to strengthen and enhance the curriculum area, increase the numbers of applicants and enrollees, and thus to ensure the administration concentration's continuing place in the school.

There are a number of confluent forces or variables that are thought to be related to the decline in the number of graduate social work students electing to concentrate in administration. These include the following: increased emphasis during the 1980s on careers that lead to increased levels of economic gain and status — for example, pursuit of a Master's in Business Administration (MBA); alternative graduate educational choices of students, for example, MSW students opting to prepare for careers in self-employed clinical practice; a deterioration of public and non-profit management salaries which has received recent federal government attention and the fact that fewer schools of social work now offer an administration major than in the past (U.S. Office of Personnel Management, 1989; Specht, 1990; CSWE, 1989). Thus, the reduction in the number of concentrations in administration is likely a direct result of reduced student demand for them, since many social work program decisions are based on enrollment figures. This reduction, in turn, closes off options for future students.

However, is the supply of professionally prepared social work administrators a result of a significant decrease in the field's demand for them? If funding for human services is any measure of the potential demand, then the answer is no. Since the mid-1960s, we have witnessed periods of incremental expansion and concentration of public funding of the human services (Levine, 1980). We are now in a period of what could be called "steady-state" public finance. As a percent of the GNP, federal spending for human services remained steady with the growth of our economy (Congressional Budget Office (CBO), 1985). Since state governments are essentially reactive to the economy, public funding has led to significant fluctuations in expansion and contraction. But it has essentially been "steady-state" in nature (CBO, 1985).

In essence, even with the reductions in funding for human services of the Reagan era, we have seen the continued, steady demand for human service administrators. Moreover, it is likely that the potential demand for professionally prepared social work administrators and human service managers will continue at a stable, if not increased, rate especially given predictions for the expansion of human services in the 1990s.

If the supply is diminishing and the demand remains stable, or even increases, how will the shortfall be met? This is the issue that the Council on Social Work Education (CSWE) and the schools of social work nationally face at this time. In the early 1970s, the rapid growth of administration concentrations in Schools of Social Work was a response to the staffing of human services agencies with MBAs, MPAs or by MSWs with clinical preparation. The principle underlying this expansion was that social agencies are best lead by professionally trained social workers who could integrate social work values with management technology and more clearly communicate this integration to other social workers in the agencies (Patti, 1984). As Teicher (1985) has said, "The ability to perform well and wisely, to steer the social agency constructively for humane purposes, is best acquired by professional social work education and experience, combined with powerful identification with social work values and ethics" (p. 44). Although the debate about who is best trained to manage human service agencies continues (Rimer, 1987; Cupaiuolo & Miringoff, 1988), most social work educators would argue in favor of leadership trained within the profession.

Ultimately, the role of social work within its service domain depends upon the profession's representation in the ranks of leaders and managers. As stated by Edwards and Gummer (1988): "If social workers are to provide the kinds of services that they see are needed by their clients and if they are to advocate for the public policy legislation and budgets to support these services, they first must regain or solidify their control over their organizational base. To do so, they must present themselves as knowledgeable and competent managers, second to none" (pp. 25-26).

For social work education, the issue of future social work administrative leadership becomes acute when schools of social work experience a decline in applications to administration concentrations. What should a school of social work do when faced with such a decline? The following is an example of how one school dealt with the issue.

STRATEGIES FOR INCREASING APPLICANT DEMAND: A CASE EXAMPLE

Background

The Administration Concentration at the University of Connecticut School of Social Work was established in 1977. For the first ten years (1977-1987), an average of twenty-five students were accepted annually into the program; the ratio of applications to students admitted ranged from 3:1 to 4:1. Of the total student body of 350-400 at the School in a given year, approximately fifty-five to sixty students are working toward an MSW with a concentration in social work administration, while another thirty to forty students have selected administration as their minor concentration. From 1977 to 1986, the years for which figures are available, 75.3 percent of administration majors were women and 21 percent were either African-American or Hispanic, close to the School's overall minority admissions rate of 23 percent. Whereas the proportions of women and minorities in the administration concentration approximate those of the total student body, a much higher proportion of administration majors pursue the degree while maintaining employment in their social agencies — 75 percent of students in administration as compared to 21 percent in casework.

Philosophy

The Administration concentration was founded on the belief that the MSW in Administration can provide optimal training for human service management. Unique among management degrees, the MSW curriculum offers a grounding in professional values and ethics; knowledge of the system of social welfare policy and services; knowledge of relevant human service technologies (Miringoff, 1980) or what is known in management circles as knowledge of the product; socialization toward a shared culture with direct service providers; and foundation knowledge of human behavior and interpersonal skills to undergird the critical human relations side of management. When merged with education on modern management techniques and traditional and new management theories within an administration concentration, the MSW provides the ingredients for effective human service management.

From the outset, faculty at the University of Connecticut designed a social work administration program that sought to balance and integrate social work values and knowledge with "state of the art" management technology. Admission to the administration sequence is limited to students who have a minimum of three years of social work experience. The integration of professional foundation and technological competence requires a fundamental educational philosophy that is expressed both in form and substance. The latter focuses on curriculum and educators who are proficient in "state of the art" management. The former requires creating a climate and educational culture in which everyone — faculty, students, field instructors and field agencies — deals with one another as professional colleagues. Personal and mutual concern, caring and respect are norms for faculty and students, in the classroom as well as in the community. Adult learning principles (Knowles, 1978) are opera-

tionalized in experiential classroom learning activities, student selected and managed projects, and in clearly articulated criteria for
evaluating student learning in both the field and the classroom.

Several years ago, in part to assist the majority of our students
who balance coursework with the demands of jobs, field placements, and family roles, faculty initiated two new course designs.
One is an intensive course, conducted on weekends. Another is a
series of one credit, two-day skill-shops devoted to "state-of-the-
art" management technology. The latter has included topics such as
staff development and training, legal issues for social work administrators, and managing change among others. These more intensive
approaches have been evaluated positively by students and faculty
and have served as models for other curriculum units in the School.

Another feature of the collegial educational culture and climate is
the continuing association between former students and the School,
which enhances both alumni professional development and the
practice relevance of the curriculum. A number of graduates of the
program have become field instructors and in a few cases, visiting
lecturers or adjunct faculty. Meetings with administration concentration field instructors each semester provide regular on-going contact with graduates and their agencies. Conferences and professional meetings are also opportunities to continue relationships with
graduates. Agency-based faculty research is aided by graduates
who hold key agency positions. Thus, we believe that the efforts to
operationalize the philosophy throughout the curriculum pay off in
terms of students' ability to integrate social work values and management technology. Empirical evidence of this in their practice
awaits future research; what we can attest to is a high level of "es-
prit de corps" among students and alumni.

Despite these positive aspects of our concentration, the facts
were clear: applications were declining. From 1984 to 1988 the
annual number of applications to administration dropped from forty
to twenty-three. This paralleled a decline in the number of students
applying to the other concentrations, particularly the "macro" concentrations, namely community organization and policy and planning. While there was an overall decline in all applications for admission to the School during this period, the decline in "macro"

concentration applications was three times as great as for the case-work and groupwork concentration (University of Connecticut School of Social Work, September 9, 1988).

Clearly, from our perspective, an aggressive approach to marketing the social work administration major was needed. At the same time, another problem was asserting itself: the increased proportion of full-time students who were already employed in management-level positions and for whom the School's requirement that one of the two required placements be outside of their agency created real problems. Thus, a series of strategies was undertaken centered around the development of student-staffed management teams.

Student-Staffed Management Consulting Team

The idea for a student-staffed management team was conceived in late spring 1988, primarily as an attempt to strengthen the field practicum component of the curriculum. Specifically, students requesting to complete the requirements for the second field placement by continuing as managers with new assignments in their own agencies were additionally required to participate in the team as a condition of faculty approval of their placement plans. The intent was to provide additional learning experiences in a new setting — the team's client organization — as well as have new collegial and leadership experiences.

Testing the concept. The first team was convened in the 1988-89 academic year. The team's client was the concentration itself, in order to provide an opportunity to test the concept of a student team "in house" before consulting with outside agencies. Moreover, there were many opportunities for developing and enhancing the concentration that faculty were anxious to pursue, including the problem of declining applications. Indeed, in an early meeting with faculty, this problem emerged and was adopted as the central focus of the team's activities during the year.

Working with one faculty member serving as team leader, the group sought first to fully define the problem. An informal needs/ issues assessment was undertaken with the following "client" groups:

1. alumni of the Administration Sequence;
2. current administration students;
3. administrators and field faculty in current and former field placements;
4. others in the community concerned about and knowledgeable in social work administration; and
5. various groups at the School including faculty, professional staff of the school's continuing education program, admissions, alumni affairs, financial aid, and grants development.

Results of the assessment identified the following issues as related to declining applications:

1. the lack of information about social work administration in general and the school's program;
2. the need for career guidance for potential applicants to the sequence; and
3. the under use of alumni as recruiters of applicants to the sequence.

From these results, the team established its overall goal: increasing applications to administration by thirty percent for the 1989-90 academic year. This goal would be achieved with two overall strategies:

1. to increase the visibility of the sequence and social work administration as a viable career choice; and
2. to improve and increase the information about the concentration that is available to prospective students.

A short-range workplan was developed which focused on a number of activities. These included the development and printing of a brochure on the administration major at the school; two recruitment breakfasts involving prospective applicants and alumni; improving the school's information sessions for prospective applicants; increasing access for preapplication advisement by sequence faculty; and a small fundraising effort to support other team activities. While minority recruitment was identified as a need, in these initial activities it was addressed through the general strategies such as ensuring attention to minority representation in the activities planned.

The team outlined a longer-range plan to increase visibility, information and financial support for prospective students. Activities in this plan included initiation of a comprehensive continuing education program in social work administration under the leadership of concentration faculty and in conjunction with the School's continuing education division; initiation of a social work administration newsletter; exploring employer-supported educational leave as an employee benefit; and exploring funding and scholarship projects that could be either school or agency-based. While the time limitations of a year-long practicum precluded this team's work on any of these longer-range activities, their suggestions are reflected in the discussion below of implications of our experience for the profession and other schools of social work.

The results of the team's effort were very positive. In 1989, applications to the administration sequence increased forty-three percent over the 1988 total. Equally important, members gave high ratings to the experience of participating on the team. Overall, they felt that they had learned a great deal about consulting, workplan and project development, and about teamwork, in particular gaining insights about specific roles each member played in achieving the project's outcomes.

Continuing pro-active outreach. The six member management consulting team for the 1989-1990 academic year built on and expanded the work of the previous year's team, particularly in its focus on increasing the visibility of the concentration. The client group focus was broadened to include all alumni of the School as well as all social work agency administrators in the New England region. The specific objectives of the team action plan were to:

1. broaden professional development opportunities for graduates who are social work administrators;
2. focus on issues and topics that represent state-of-the-art social work administration; and
3. expand the School's recruitment of social work administration students.

To achieve these objectives the team decided to initiate what is hoped will become an annual event: a professional development state-of-the-art management workshop. The title of the first workshop was "Image management for social work organizations: Building block for the future." The lead speaker was a nationally known figure in the field and the workshop was well received.

Results

These events and activities have achieved, in a small way, some positive results for the administration concentration at the University of Connecticut School of Social Work. Specifically, we increased applications for 1989-90 year; the visibility of administration has been increased; we have come to recognize two of our important resources—alumni and current students—and to better utilize their commitment to the program; and we have enhanced the field practicum for some employed second year students. More importantly, the experience has helped to underscore the continuing challenges of promoting and ensuring the education of social work administrators. These challenges are outlined below, followed by recommendations for individual schools and the profession for meeting them.

THE CHALLENGES AND THEIR IMPLICATIONS

The Challenges

There are at least five key challenges that the profession and individual schools of social work must be prepared to meet if the number of social-work trained administrators in the human services is to increase. These are delineated briefly below:

1. The profession must make a commitment to training its own leadership; administration concentrations in schools of social work cannot be solely at the mercy of uninformed student demand.
2. More information about career opportunities in social work administration is needed. Neither the option of an administration major in social work, nor its unique curriculum, as de-

scribed earlier, is well-known among applicants to schools of social work.

3. In line with the above, the profession — and in particular, schools of social work — must aggressively market the unique quality of social work administration. Neugeboren (1990) identifies this uniqueness as substantive knowledge in four major areas: (1) a field of practice; (2) service delivery technologies; (3) community; and (4) human relations skills.

4. The vast majority of human service managers are professionally prepared in other disciplines or have an MSW in clinical practice with no management training. We believe neither group is adequately prepared for administering social work agencies which requires the ability to integrate social work values and knowledge with modern management technology. The image (including earning opportunities) of the social work-trained administrator held by potential applicants, funders and personnel committees must be enhanced to enable the MSW to offer an attractive alternative to the MBA and MPA for leadership positions in social agencies. Moreover, if we are to maintain these positions for the social work profession, a major national thrust in post-Master's training for non-managerial (clinically trained) MSWs is needed.

5. Most students, particularly those already in administrative positions, must fund graduate training with their own earnings. Moreover, they are understandably reluctant to leave their jobs (particularly where seniority is concerned) for the field placement. Increased flexibility in work-study arrangements may be needed in schools of social work as well as encouragement for agencies — in particular public agencies — to develop and maintain these programs. The needs are great for increased stipends, fellowships, paid leaves and other supports as well as creatively developed and structured practica.

Recommendations to Schools of Social Work

Based on our assessment of the problem of declining interest in social work administration and on our attempts to increase the number of applicants in administration at our school, we would like to offer two sets of recommendations.

The first, offered to schools of social work, is based on the surprising degree of success that some of our relatively low-effort activities generated. Locally held information and recruitment breakfasts were particularly effective. Alumni were asked to bring at least one colleague potentially interested in social work administration to the session. Prospects were reached directly and personally. A number of people had questions over career directions and benefitted from the opportunity to hear about macro practice and the educational program in administration. Alumni involvement, in this and other activities, is another key. Neugeboren (1990) describes a one-credit career development course to help students market their skills in social work administration.

Second, in re-establishing or preserving a concentration in social work administration, institutional commitment to its survival is essential. Clearly, one reason why our school's administration program survived long enough to undertake this project is our system of admissions quotas by concentration, and maintenance of these quotas even when applicant-acceptance ratios have differed across concentrations. Thus, the administration concentration has twenty places in each first year class even if our acceptance ratio falls to 1.5 : 1 while in casework sequence only 1 out of 3 or 4 applicants is accepted. This requires a willingness to allocate educational resources on the basis of needs of the profession rather than solely in response to applicant demand. Introducing this idea into discussion at other schools is important as part of any overall strategy to increase the numbers of trained administrators.

Recommendations to the Profession

In addition to these strategies for individual schools, we recommend that a national program be defined and implemented, led by the Association on Community Organization and Social Administration (ACOSA), in collaboration with the National Network for Social Work Managers and the National Association of Social Workers (NASW) to include the following three major strategies:

1. Conducting a national survey of schools of social work and selected social agencies to determine the scope of the problems described above and to detail successful strategies undertaken to deal with them.

2. Documenting, publishing, and disseminating the results of the above survey to all schools of social work.
3. Developing and undertaking a national program of "image enhancement" of social work administration/management through the collaborative efforts of CSWE, ACOSA, the National Association of Social Workers (NASW), and the National Network of Social Work Managers in the areas of recruitment, professional development, and salary enhancement.

Recruitment

More than ever, young people are seeking challenging careers. Whether we stimulate those about to choose a career or attract people now in the human services to prepare themselves professionally for administrative positions, there is a need for a nationally coordinated recruitment of the best qualified candidates to enter the ranks of human services management. While the values of power, position, and money will continue to attract many of the best minds in our nation, increasingly other more altruistic values will attract people seeking more meaning to life in a so-called money society. The continued popularity of the Peace Corps is proof of such appeal. If fashioned, packaged, and marketed by image enhancement professionals, such a national recruitment effort can be successful. It would require strong ACOSA-CSWE leadership in close partnership with all Schools of Social Work, NASW and the National Network. Such an effort would also require public-private partnerships, probably with foundation support.

Moreover, a major emphasis is needed to recruit multicultural applicants. Social work has had a value commitment to equal opportunity and advancement for minorities and women. Statistics on characteristics of managers, however, show that whites, especially white males, still predominate in top positions in social agencies (Ewalt, 1987). Now, the demographic imperative can be added to the value commitment to convince us of the necessity to attract more minorities, "new Americans," and women to leadership positions (Weil, 1989). The pool of new job entrants will continue to grow increasingly female, hispanic, black and immigrant (Butz and others, 1982). According to Johnston and Packer (1987), between now and the year 2000, eighty percent of new job entrants will be women, minorities, and immigrants. Without aggressive and imaginative outreach to these groups, truly attracting the "best and brightest" will not be possible. In addition, schools should work together to develop curricula which will prepare students for managing diversity in a way which maximizes the dynamic and creative potential of the increasingly diverse workforce.

Professional Development

A large number of social work administrators and human services managers have educational preparation in other disciplines, or have clinical-casework backgrounds and little formal management education. Numerous schools of social work have, from time to time, tried to address the issue of professional development for the social work administrator/practitioner. However, there has never been a systematic national effort to deal with this issue. We propose a national professional certificate program in social work administration developed and implemented under the leadership of ACOSA in concert with CSWE, NASW, and the National Network. The curriculum would be competency-based with a nationally recognized certificate awarded upon completion of the program.

Salary Enhancement

Social work professionals, with strong NASW support, have expended great effort to have third party payments legitimated for MSW clinicians. This effort has been driven by both professional and economic reasons. An equal effort needs to be invested in increasing remuneration for all social workers, particularly for social work administrators. Professionals in all fields pursue administrative positions in part because the remuneration is the highest in the organization. However, compared to administrative careers in business or public administration, or in education and health such a career in social work is less financially attractive. The depressed nature of social work administrative salaries has a direct and significant effect on the rate of applications to administration concentrations in schools of social work. Thus, as part of the image enhancement strategy, it is vital that a major effort be made to significantly upgrade the salaries of social work administrators.

The strategies presented here are among the many possible ap-

proaches to increasing the number of social work trained administrators. Others could include a re-examination of the curriculum
policy statement (CSWE, 1982), particularly its assumptions about
essential curriculum content and structure; and the establishment of
a national fellowship program to develop and support challenging
and prominent field placements in management.

CONCLUSION

This article presented some of the current issues in social work
administration. Problems about declining enrollment and a reduction in the number of schools offering a concentration in administration as well as some of the strategies for dealing with these problems may have relevance for other macro concentrations such as
community organizing, policy, and planning. As a profession, we
must take action if social workers are to achieve and maintain their
place as leaders of tomorrow's ever more complex human services
organizations. While we might focus our concern and attention on
the current reduction of societal investment in human services, of
equal concern is the significant improvement and modernization in
their management. Social work educators must take the lead,
through their professional organizations, to ensure that the "best"
and the "brightest" are attracted to careers in social work administration and are able to develop leadership competence in high quality graduate social work programs.

REFERENCES

Butz, W.P., McCarthy, K.F.; Morrison, P.A. & Vaieana, M.E. Demographic
    challenges in America's future. In U.S. Catholic Conference, *America: Immi-
    gration, refugees, population and our future*, Washington, DC, 1982.
Congressional Budget Office. *Reducing the deficit: Spending and revenue op-
    tions*. Washington, DC: Author, February 1985.
Council on Social Work Education. *Statistics on social work education in the
    United States*. Washington, DC: CSWE, 1989.
Cupaiuolo, A.A. & Miringoff, M.L. MBA, MPA, MSW: Is there a degree of
    choice for human service management? In P.R. Keys and L.H. Ginsberg
    (Eds.), *New management in human services*. Silver Spring, MD: NASW,
    1988.
Edwards, R.L., & Gummer, B. Management of social services: Current perspec-

tives and future trends. In P.R. Keys & L.H. Ginsberg (Eds.), *New management in human services*. Silver Spring, MD: NASW, 1988.

Ewalt, P. Women in social work administration. Paper presented at the CSWE Annual Program Meeting, St. Louis, March 1987.

Healy, L.M., Pine, B.A. & Weiner, M.E. *Social work leadership for human services management in the 1990s: The challenge of the new demographic reality*. West Hartford, CT: University of Connecticut School of Social Work, 1989.

Johnston, W.B. and Packer, A.E. *Workforce 2000: Work and workers for the 21st century*. Indianapolis, IN: Hudson Institute, 1987.

Knowles, M. *The adult learner: A neglected species* (2nd ed.). Houston, TX: Gulf, 1978.

Levine, Charles H. *Managing fiscal stress*. Chatham, NJ: Chatham House, 1980.

Miringoff, M.L. *Management in human service organizations*. New York: Macmillan, 1980.

Neugeboren, B. Career development in social work administration. *Administration in Social Work*, 1990, *14*(1), 47-63.

Patti, R. Who leads the human services? The prospects for social work leadership in an age of political conservatism. *Administration in Social Work*, 1984, *9*(1), 17-29.

Rimer, E. Social administration education: Reconceptualizing the conflict with MPA, MBA, and MPH programs. *Administration in Social Work*, 1987, *11*(2), 45-55.

Specht, H. Social work and the popular psychotherapies. *Social Service Review*, 1990, *64*(3), 345-357.

Teicher, M.I. Who should manage a social agency? In S. Slavin (Ed.), *An introduction to human services management*, Vol. I. New York: The Haworth Press, 1985.

United States Office of Personnel Management. *Report of the national commission on public service*. Washington, DC, April 1989.

University of Connecticut School of Social Work. *Final admissions report*. West Hartford, 1988.

University of Connecticut School of Social Work. Field Education Statistics. West Hartford, 1990.

Weil, M. Gender and ethnic shifts: managing for leadership development and responses to changing client populations. In L.M. Healy et al. *Social work leadership for human services management in the 1990s: The challenge of the new demographic reality*. West Hartford, CT: University of Connecticut School of Social Work, 1989.

Political Activism in Social Work: A Study of Social Work Educators

Nancy L. Mary, DSW
Claudia Webb Ellano, MSW
Jean Newell, BSW

INTRODUCTION

In spite of the national emergence of baccalaureate programs and the growth of both master's and doctoral education in social work, social work education is approaching the 1990s unprepared in the political arena. Although the National Association of Social Workers increased its awareness of the connection between social work and political activity, through the development of ELAN (Education Legislation Action Network) and PACE (Political Action for Candidate Endorsement), social work classroom and field curricula do not reflect this awareness.

The drive toward specialization has created concentrations to meet the needs of new constituents, e.g., occupational social work. But as the federal response to social needs continues to wane and the emphasis on private/public collaboration increases, the development of political skills and experiences to help society attain greater social justice is not a high priority for most social work educators.

Dr. Mary is Assistant Professor, Social Work Department, California State University-San Bernardino, 5500 University Parkway, San Bernardino, CA 92407. Ms. Ellano is Service Chief, Older Adult Services Orange County Health Care Agency, Costa Mesa, CA, and a faculty member at California State University, Long Beach, Department of Social Work. Ms. Newell is an Associate of "Network," Washington, DC.

An earlier version of this paper was presented at the Association on Community Organization and Social Administration Symposium, Annual Program Meeting, Council on Social Work Education, Chicago, 1989.

Haynes and Mickelson's (1985) survey of 25% of all graduate and undergraduate bulletins for social work programs lends evidence to the low level of commitment toward the teaching of political content. Only 6 out of 122 courses surveyed across HBSE, Practice, Research, and Social Policy curriculum areas, contained titles or descriptions reflecting political content or terminology. This inattention in the formal curriculum to the means of social change in terms of knowledge and skills of the political process is problematic if members of the profession are committed to the goal of social reform.

Webster defines partisan broadly as "a firm adherent to a party, faction, cause, or person." Mahaffey (1987, p. 285) states that politics involves "seeking power, exercising power and achieving compromise when appropriate" (p. 285). Political activity includes political involvement beyond voting. For the purpose of this study, it encompasses such behaviors as discussion of public issues, belonging to political organizations, written or verbal communications with public officials, campaign activities, and political contributions (Wolk, 1981).

SOCIAL WORKERS AND POLITICAL ACTION: A BRIEF HISTORY

Since its inception, social work has involved a struggle between function and cause, between commitment to the individual and public responsibility, between the world of the clinician and the sociopolitical arena. The 1920s represented a paradox in social welfare and social reform. While the American Association of Social Workers (AASW) focused on the establishment of professional standards in practice and training for this young profession, the 1920s — a decade of prosperity — was a time for planting new seeds of social reconstruction that anticipated much of the New Deal (Chambers, 1963; Leiby, 1978).

During the pre-Roosevelt period from 1929 to 1933, New York social workers, alarmed by unemployment rates, worked with three governors on welfare reform. While settlement house workers attended Senate hearings on unemployment and lobbied for Federal assistance to supplement the relief funds of local governments, others, such as Mary Van Kleeck of the Russell Sage Foundation, suggested a more radical reconstruction of social and economic institutions.

At the 1934 conference of AASW, the first national meeting of the profession to discuss collective political action, delegates raised important issues with respect to programs and social reforms that social workers should support. Conflict between moderate and radical viewpoints rose in strength at the 1934 National Conference of Social Work, with the rank and file movement stressing broad social change based on a union model, and a more moderate concern that the association limit itself to consensus areas such as professional standards and the adequacy of relief measures (Leighninger, 1987).

With the termination of the Federal Emergency Relief Administration in 1935, social workers still pushed for more adequate public relief. Strategies differed, however. The rank and file contingent engaged in mass protests with labor and the unemployed, while the moderate majority of AASW pursued an advisory role in public policy making. In 1937-1938 a gradual retreat from political activity occurred, as attention was turned to professional staffing of the Social Security programs and psychotherapeutic models of casework in child and family agencies (Day, 1989).

The profession's focus, during the 1940s, was the relationship between the social sciences and social work practice. How to develop and maintain professional autonomy, while at the same time using sound interdisciplinary theories from biology, psychology, sociology, and anthropology, was the challenge of interdisciplinary social work projects at Western Reserve's School of Applied Social Sciences (SASS) and the interdisciplinary faculty seminar at the University of Michigan (Leighninger, 1987). These efforts, alongside the developing specialized professional groups such as the American Association of Group Workers and the Association for the Study of Community Organization, represented a continued debate around social work as a method, a craft, and a science, a debate with ramifications for the proper arenas of social work.

The 1950s saw a more cautious approach to the political involvement of social workers. The major purpose of the then new National Association of Social Workers was to enhance professional status, with emphasis placed on high standards and training, rather than political action. Even the social action stance envisioned by some in the early NASW years focused on a social planning model over a more adversarial political organizing approach.

The War on Poverty, Civil Rights Movement, and outcry for "citizen participation" of the 1960s shook social workers into another re-examination of their role in social action and politics. Some from within and without the profession called for social workers to engage in both lobbying as well as formal involvement in a political party structure (Schneiderman, 1970; Ribicoff, 1962). Others emphasized the political role of social work from within the profession's framework for community organization (Thurz, 1966). Brager's (1968) work with the Community Organization Curriculum Development Project of Columbia outlined the necessity for political behavior, and the knowledge of power and skills of manipulation as part of the role of social worker as advocate. This work was influential in NASW's 1969 adoption of advocacy as an approved social work role.

As a profession, the NASW took a more active role during the Kennedy-Johnson era around the Social Security Amendments, the War on Poverty and the Civil Rights Movement. Local chapters were allowed to endorse local, and later national candidates for election, and coalitions were formed with such groups as the National Welfare Rights Organization.

But as the War on Poverty wound down, and the Vietnam War escalated, the mid-seventies began to see social workers most comfortable with consultant roles and emphasis on individually focused change agent approaches (Leighninger, 1987). Community organizing lost its momentum as macro-practice modes such as administration and social planning moved to the forefront. The 1980s saw massive growth in the federal deficit, in low wage employment with the continued application of the "trickle down" response to poverty, and, in general, heightened apathy toward social problems as evidenced by lower voter participation.

Piven and Cloward (1988), fearing the Republican/corporate mobilization symbolized by Reagan's election in 1980, formed Human SERVE in 1983 to persuade private, voluntary agencies to make nonpartisan voter registration services available at their reception desks in order to build long-term electoral resistance to slashes in the social programs. Few voluntary agencies participated, however.[1] But the split in social work focus continued, with a growing professional political arm (PACE) alongside a burgeoning move of NASW members toward private (clinical) practice.

Indeed, the tensions surrounding the role of social work and social action are alive today. The extent to which the profession is committed to public service vs. private practice and the emphasis on a clinical knowledge base vs. skill building in negotiation, lobbying, and brokering as part of policy-making are some of the current debates. And the question remains: "What is the role and obligation of social workers in political action?"

POLITICAL INVOLVEMENT IN THE GENERAL POPULATION

Given the aforementioned definition, by Wolk, of political participation as a variety of activities along a continuum, Woodward and Roper (1950), in their seminal work on political participation among Americans, characterized 73% of the population as politically "inert" while only 10% of the adult population were "very active." The remaining 17% fell somewhere in between.

Milbrath (1965) summarized findings of previous research, up to that time, on political activity in the United States in a similar manner: 60% play largely "spectator" roles in the political process; "they watch, they cheer, they vote, but they do not battle." Only one to two percent could be called "gladiators." Gladiators not only participate in the above activities, but are also "drawn into the political fray; they attend meetings, campaign, become active in a party, solicit money, run for and hold public and party office." Those who make a transition from spectator to gladiator are the "transitionals"; those who participate in a wider repertoire of political acts, such as making monetary contributions to candidates and attending political meetings.

Milbrath points out, in addition, that a cumulative hierarchy of political involvement has been evidenced in research (Almond & Verba, 1963); that is, persons who engage in topmost political behavior such as holding public office, are very likely to perform behaviors lower in rank, e.g., wearing a political button or sticker on their car. The obverse does not hold true, however. Minimally involved persons confine their actions to those acts ranking low in the hierarchy.

Verba, Nie, and Kim (1978), in a survey of political participation across several nations, developed a broader hierarchy of participation variables ranging from contact with a local official on a personal problem to working for a political party. They found clear clusters of activities, in each of the nations surveyed, similar to those in Milbrath's (1965) hierarchy of political involvement.

SOCIAL WORK AND POLITICS

Wolk's 1981 survey of 470 members of the Michigan Chapter of NASW regarding their political involvement supported Milbrath's earlier finding that the nature of political activity is hierarchical. However, Wolk's sample of social workers was more politically active than the general populations studied by Woodward and Roper (1950) and by Milbrath (1965). For example, 45% of social workers were classified as "active" as opposed to 17% of the general population in the Woodward and Roper study.

Wolk (1981), Milbrath (1965), and Woodward and Roper (1950) all examined the impact of demographic variables on political participation. No significant relationships were found between levels of political involvement and race or educational level. Milbrath's work with the general population concluded that men were more likely to participate in political activity than women, but that this sexual gap might be narrowing with changing economic and social trends. However, both Wolk and Woodward and Roper reported that trends indicated females were more likely than males to be politically active, though differences were not statistically significant.

Income levels consistently influenced political involvement in these studies. All three of the above mentioned studies found a positive relationship between political activity and increased income. With respect to the variable of age, Milbrath (1965) found that political participation among the general population rose gradually as age increased, then peaked and leveled off in the 40s and 50s; involvement then declined above age 60. Wolk's (1981) study of social workers and Woodward and Roper's (1950) general population study both reported increases in political participation with age; however, no levelling off occurred above age 60.

POLITICAL INVOLVEMENT AND SOCIAL WORK VALUES

Social workers were reminded, over 40 years ago, that "social work, in principle and in tenet, is not separable from social reform; the very nature of the objectives of social work as well as its role in a democratic society, commits it to working for the betterment of social living for all people" (Howard, 1954, p. 159). If social work and politics are congruent, they will share a set of philosophical value assumptions.

In an examination of social work values, Abbott (1988) constructed a Professional Opinion Scale, using values in the NASW Public Social Policy Statements; the Scale contained four value dimensions: (1) respect for basic rights, (2) sense of social responsibility, (3) commitment to individual freedom, and (4) support of self-determination. Her findings, from a sample of members of seven major professions, revealed that members of different groups do have different value preferences, with social workers presenting the strongest degree of concurrence with these four values.

In a comparison of a 1968 survey (Epstein, 1969) and one done in 1984 (Reeser, 1986), Reeser and Epstein (1987) focused more specifically on views toward social action. In their look at social work attitudes toward poverty, activist strategies, and commitment to activist goals, their findings suggested significant changes since the 1960s. Social workers in 1968 reported greater commitment to involvement in social change and an activist goal-orientation than those in the 1984 study. Respondents, in 1984, were less likely to regard the elimination of poverty as a goal or to endorse an activist goal orientation. However, both groups preferred non-controversial "consensus" strategies over tactics such as social protest.

Haynes and Mickelson (1991) have asserted that, for the most part, social workers have overtly disagreed with a view of the inherently political nature of their work; the majority have believed that social work is and should be apolitical. Haynes and Mickelson (1986) point out also that social values, for example self-determination of an individual and an organization, appear to be incongruent between the micro- and macro-levels of practice:

> Social workers too often have acted as if budgets and fiscal considerations were not only inconsequential to their programs but also as if such considerations were inhumane. .... Social workers must learn that there is no incompatibility between caring, competence, and humanitarianism, on the one hand, and fiscal efficiency on the other. (p. 16)

Nancy Humphreys (1988) remarked that there is the image that social workers are contaminated once they enter politics. She concluded that the profession accepts the legislative advocacy role of the social worker but balks at the "insider" roles of being a campaign worker or on the staff of an elected official. And, overall, social workers have some discomfort with the "co-mingling" of partisan politics and social work.

Daniel Thurz, writing in 1966 as the Associate Director of VISTA (Volunteers in Service to America), asserted that social work and social action were, indeed, congruent. Thurz identified three assumptions which underlie social work and social action. The first is that "social action is the business of social work." The second is that conflict is necessary and can be constructive. Thurz' third proposition is that social work cannot be wholly scientific. This includes the tenet that values judgments are part of social work practice—that to "bury one's head in the sand and pretend a detachment" (p. 14) or a disinterested point of view may be unreal and self-defeating.

THE STUDY OF SOCIAL WORK EDUCATORS

The Research Questions

The two areas of the present investigation focused on the level of political involvement of social workers and their perceived value conflicts regarding social work and politics. The first area of investigation included the following questions: What is the level of political involvement of social work faculty and field instructors? Are demographic variables related to the level and types of political activity engaged in by social work faculty and field instructors?

Value conflicts are the focus of the second area under examination. To what extent do social work field instructors and faculty agree with Thurz' value assumptions? These assumptions are: social work is social action; conflict is a necessary ingredient in social work; and decisions in social work cannot be value free.

Methodology

Data were gathered on political involvement using an expanded version of Milbrath's (1965) hierarchy of political behavior. Respondents were asked to indicate with a "yes" or "no" whether they had ever engaged in various political activities ranging from "Have you ever worn a button or put a political sticker on your car?" to "Have you ever been elected to public office?"

The hierarchy is constructed with the assumption that time and energy reflect personal commitment and are variables that define the extent of one's political involvement; thus time and energy costs are least for the activities at the bottom of the list of the hierarchy, and highest for the activities at the top.

Milbrath then categorized these behaviors as "spectator," "transitional" and "gladiator" level behaviors, the validity of which is based on percentages of Americans who have engaged in particular activities in studies done by Campbell et al. (1960), Lane (1959), and Woodward and Roper (1950). These categories were expanded by the present researchers through the addition of fifteen items, creating a hierarchy of a total of twenty-seven political behaviors.

It was the hypothesis of the researchers that faculty and field instructors whose primary area of practice/instruction was macro-level change would be involved in political activities to a greater degree than those whose primary focus was micro (direct) practice.

The second area of investigation—respondents' perceptions of compatibility between socialwork values and politics—was made through a series of belief statements based on Thurz' three assumptions regarding social work and social action. Respondents were asked to rate the statements on a four point Likert scale from "strongly agree" to "strongly disagree." For example: "Social work, in principle, is not separable from social reform."

The Sample

Anonymous questionnaires were mailed to 50 faculty of a large urban university, including both part and full time faculty in both BSW and MSW programs. The survey was conducted in late Spring, 1988. One hundred and ninety-five field instructors, in agencies located in two urban counties of Southern California, were surveyed; the agencies ranged from battered womens' shelters to public welfare agencies. Field instructors supervised both undergraduate and graduate students.

A mailing of 245 questionnaires yielded a response of 129 completed surveys. A response rate of 53% was obtained (23 faculty, 104 field instructors, 2 unidentified). As the response rate was moderate for a mailed questionnaire, no follow up efforts were made to increase the number of responses. No data were collected on nonrespondents. Profile demographics were collected such as race, sex, and income, as well as other variables such as practice setting, number of years in practice, and primary practice method of the respondent.

Data were analyzed primarily in terms of frequencies and percentiles, examination of means and cross tabulations of involvement scores and demographic variables.

RESULTS

Two-thirds of the respondents were between the ages of 36 and 55, with 3 to 14 years of practice experience. Thirty-two percent (41) were male and sixty-two percent (80) female; 8 did not indicate their sex. The ethnic breakdown was: 66% White, 10% Black, 9% Asian, 7% Hispanic, 1% American Indian; 7% did not indicate ethnicity.

Field instructors' agencies represented an equal private/public mix, the majority (70%) having spent the major portion of their practice in the fields of mental health, children and youth, or health and medical settings. Three-quarters of the respondents held an

MSW as their highest degree. Seven percent (9) had doctorates in social work. Two percent (3) had a BSW degree. Eight percent (11) had a BA or MA in another field, and 8% (11) had other unspecified degrees.

About three-quarters of field instructors supervised MSW students and one-fifth supervised BSW students; 7% (8) supervised both levels of students.

Political Involvement

Table 1 shows the percentage of both field instructors and faculty who had ever engaged in various political activities.

Findings by both Wolk (1981) and the present study indicate a greater degree of political involvement of social workers compared to Milbraith's general population studies. Wolk's study and that of Woodward and Roper used somewhat different scales; thus, cross-study comparisons of "active" and "inactive" involvement are difficult to make. Notable in this study are significantly large social worker contributions of time and money to political campaigns, caucuses and candidates, as well as some of the "spectator" activities such as voting and engaging in political discussions. In only two areas were there significant differences between faculty and field instructors: faculty were more apt to work in a political action group to do community problem solving, and more apt to testify before a legislative committee, than were field instructors.

Age and salary were the only factors which consistently influenced involvement in Milbrath (1965), Woodward and Roper (1950), Wolk (1981), and in the present study. A total political involvement score was constructed by summing scores for each of the political activities listed in Table 1. These scores were then grouped into "low" (0-10) and "high" (11-25) and cross-tabulated with age groupings of "under 35," "36-45" and "over 45." A significantly larger number of 36-45 year olds were politically active than those in the under 35 or over 45 age groupings ($\times 2 = 20.9$, df = 2, p < .01). Similarly, Milbrath's study of the general population found political activity peaking at age 45 and levelling off in the above 45 groups. This is not consistent with Wolk's (1981) study of social workers, nor with Woodward and Roper's

TABLE 1

Percentage of Field Instructors and Faculty
Who Had Ever Engaged in Various
Political Activities (%) n=127

Political Activity	Faculty and Field Instructors	Fac	Fld	t	General Pop.[1]
Gladiator Activities					
Been elected to a public office*	2	4	1	NS	<1
Been appointed to public office	6	15	5	NS	
Been a candidate for public ofc*	2	0	2		
Solicited political funds*	23	30	22	NS	<1
Attended a political caucus*	25	26	24	NS	4-5
Contributed time to a political campaign*	49	52	48	NS	4-5
Worked actively in a local political action group to do community problem solving	32	48	29	3.13	.08
Transitional Activities					
Made a monetary contribution to a party or candidate*	72	74	72	NS	10
Wrote a letter to a public official or candidate	77	74	79	NS	
Visited a public official or candidate*	61	74	59	NS	13
Done door-to-door or telephone canvassing	43	43	42	NS	
Been arrested for a political action	2	0	3	NS	
Circulated a petition*	56	48	58	NS	
Attended a political meeting or rally*	70	74	70	NS	
Attended a boycott, sit-in, march, demonstration	53	48	55	NS	
Testified before a legislative committee	19	30	16	2.81	.09
Testified before a community hearing (local or national)	31	35	30	NS	
Written a letter to a newspaper, magazine or journal about a political issue	29	35	27	NS	

Spectator Activities

Worn a button or put a political sticker on your car*	58	61	58	NS	15
Attempted to talk another person into voting a certain way*	69	65	70	NS	25-30
Initiated a political discussion	81	87	80	NS	
Voted for national or state officials* (on a regular basis)	89	87	89	NS	40-70
Voted for local offices and initiatives* (regularly)	89	87	89	NS	40-70
Had your name included on campaign literature as a supporter	21	35	18	NS	
Displayed a candidate's sign on your property	24	35	22	NS	
Displayed a sign supporting or opposing a proposition on your property	15	17	15	NS	
Had your name included on literature supporting or opposing a community issue	23	30	21	NS	

1
Findings from Milbraith (1965)
*these are Milbrath's items
** p< .10

(1950) study of the general populations, both of which found political involvement increased with age. Salaries were grouped as "$30,000 or less," "$30-40,000" and "above $40,000." Those making $40,000 and above were more active than those making between $30 and $40,000, with the under $30,000 group much less likely to be active ($x2 = 5.80$, df = 2, $p < .05$). This is consistent with the three previous studies cited.

Consistent with Wolk (1981), no significant differences were found in cross tabulations between political involvement and sex ($x2 = .03$, df = 1, $p = .84$), race ($x2 = 3.81$, df = 4, $p = .43$) or years of practice experience ($x2 = 4.09$, df = 3, $p = .25$). A trend existed in the latter variable, with those having the most years of experience ("15-27 or more") reporting the highest levels of political activity.

In addition, Wolk (1981) found that workers from macro levels of practice tended to be more politically active than those in direct service. Using the same fields of practice as Wolk, the present study evidenced a similar finding. When direct service and supervision were grouped together as micro-practice and all other methods were grouped as macro-practice (i.e., consultation, community organization, administration, planning and teaching) significantly higher political involvement scores were found among the latter group ($x2 = 4.47$, df $= 1$, $p < .03$).

Ideology of Politics and Social Work

The results of this area of investigation are summarized in Table 2. Responses of faculty and field instructors were combined, as little difference was found between the responses of these two groups.

Contrary to Haynes and Mickelson's (1986) assertion that social workers are apolitical, both faculty and field instructors responded in moderate agreement to the first of Thurz' three principles, that is, that social action is the business of social work. The fifth statement is the exception. While there is moderate to high agreement with the more abstract, theoretical statements, fewer respondents agreed with the necessity of attending first to the direct service needs of the client.

Respondents are less in agreement with the second assumption that social work involves value judgments (the second set of five statements). In the context of client self-determination, the majority of respondents recognized that their influence upon client decision making was not value free; similarly 60% indicated that social work does not operate apart from various political interest groups. There is more of an even split, however, when social workers were asked to respond to the more hypothetical questions regarding emotional neutrality and non-partisanship.

There was less consensus on the items measuring respondents' beliefs about the role of conflict in social work. Mixed responses occurred with regard to the role of conflict in social work and politics. And much indecision was reported with respect to the "business" and appropriate strategies of social work vs. politics.

TABLE 2

Percentage Agreement with Various Statements
About Political Activity Among Social Workers
(N= 129)

Assumption #1: Social Action/Social Work Congruence	Agree and Strongly Agree	Disagree and Strongly Disagree	Undecided
As a social worker, to effectively access resources for one's clientele one must have some understanding of political systems.	93%	5%	2%
Social work, in principle, is not separable from social reform.	82%	12%	6%
Part of a social worker's ethical responsibility to society involves engaging in political activities.	70%	21%	9%
Social work is inherently political.	67%	24%	9%
As a direct service practitioner I must always attend to the needs of my client before I engage in larger reform or political issues.	43%	47%	10%

Assumption #2:

Value Free Social Work

	Agree and Strongly Agree	Disagree and Strongly Disagree	Undecided
Because we hold high the principle of self-determination, our influence upon a client's decision making is always value free.	17%	75%	8%
Social work's professional norms make it autonomous--set it apart--from various political interest groups.	26%	59%	15%
One danger of furthering one's political involvement as a social worker is the development of a partisan position on human problems.	32%	54%	14%
Whether we work with a family, testify in court, or attend a strategy meeting, social workers should remain as emotionally neutral as possible.	39%	53%	8%
To be an effective social worker one must be politically non-partisan.	39%	53%	8%

TABLE 2 (continued)

Assumption #3:

Conflict , Social Work and
Politics

Confrontation, struggle and conflict are inherent in social work practice.	86%	9%	5%
Conflict, in all areas of social work, is necessary and can be constructive.	51%	39%	10%
Political activity by its nature always involves conflict.	47%	48%	5%
The "business" of politics is compromise; the "business" of social work is the establishment of consensus through the problem solving process.	40%	36%	24%
Social work strategy begins with an aim for consensus before resorting to confrontation; political activity begins with confrontation and to some extent stays there.	22%	53%	25%

All of the statements in Table 2 were then examined for differences between faculty and field value perspectives, as well as against the demographic variables of age, sex, race, and primary method of practice (direct vs. indirect). It was assumed that daily experiences with clients in the role of practitioner might give field instructors a different view from professors of the congruence between social work and politics or the role of conflict in social work.

With the four point Likert scale of "strongly agree" to "strongly disagree" treated as a continuous variable with "undecided" placed in the middle of the continuum, only one significant difference occurred in the mean scores of faculty and field instructors. Faculty more often agreed with the premise that "political activity by its nature always involves conflict" (Fac X = 3.6; Field X = 2.9; t = 6.36, df = 1, p < .01).

There were no trends among these statements related to race, method of practice, or age. Males, however, agreed more often than did females that the needs of clients should be attended to before engaging in larger reform or political issues (M X = 3.3;

F X = 2.8; t = 3.75, df = 1, p < .05). Slight trends indicated that males tended to see social work as more "inherently political" than did females (M X = 3.8; F X = 3.4; t = 2.79, df = 1, p < .09) and saw "political activity by nature always involving conflict" more often than did females (M X = 3.4; F X = 3.0; t = 2.77, df = 1, p < .09).

Females, on the other hand, tended to lean more toward "emotional neutrality"; females agreed more often than males that whether working with a family or in a strategy meeting, social workers "should remain emotionally neutral" (M X = 2.5; F X = 3.0; t = 3.21, df = 1, p < .07).

DISCUSSION

The researchers were heartened to see the degree to which both groups reported involvement in political activities. One-half had given time and money to a political campaign. Overall scores were consistent with Wolk (1981), showing a much higher degree of involvement of social workers than that reported by Milbrath (1965) in general population studies. Nor was it surprising that macro social workers had significantly higher levels of political activity than did direct service practitioners or supervisors.

Value conflicts did occur, most often in relation to the concepts of "impartiality" and "conflict." Social workers in the study were aware of the influence they have on clients' decision making, but whether social work operates as an interest group or involves taking partisan positions is a controversial question. There is evidence of mixed reactions, as well, to conflict and whether it is an element in politics or a necessary ingredient in social work.

Limitations of Methodology

Mention should be made of the limitations of Milbraith's measure of time and energy in a hierarchy of political activities as a valid measure of political involvement. Self-reported behavior may be less accurate than direct observation. As critical, is the lack of a cumulative history of the subject's involvement; respondents who may have written only one letter in their lifetime are as politically involved, according to this measure, as those who write weekly letters to public officials.

Sampling bias may be an issue here as well. It is conceivable that the 47% who did not return the questionnaire did not do so because of disagreement with or lack of interest in the topic. Generalizability of findings may be limited also. Although the results are consistent with Wolk's (1981) study, the sample is more narrowly drawn from an urban, Southern California population of social workers and may not adequately represent the population nationwide. For example, 45% of respondents' workplaces were either mental health or medical settings; this may not mirror more rural, less populated areas of the country.

IMPLICATIONS FOR SOCIAL WORK EDUCATION AND THE PROFESSION

The results of this study have implications for curriculum development as well as the profession as a whole. With respect to social work education, the authors recommend greater attention to the teaching of skills such as conflict resolution and confrontation within micro and macro contexts. "Power to the politician is personality to the clinician" (Humphreys, 1988). Students need to understand the role of power in human behavior, social policy, and the practice world. Knowledge and skills in brokering, negotiation and arbitration, consensus-building, and problem solving need to be introduced as tools for empowering individuals, groups, their communities and the profession. This study indicates that social workers have some ambivalence toward conflict. Appropriate learning opportunities, then, should be provided in the classroom and field that engage students in confrontation, the taking of partisan positions, influencing various constituencies, and managing adversarial relationships.

The biased nature of social work needs to be explored in the field and classroom. Social workers constitute a political interest group. Social work values, by definition, are more often associated with a democratic and humanistic agenda. One challenge of social work educators is to impart these values within a framework of critical thinking such that students arrive at partisan positions congruent with social work values, *via* a process of thoughtful examination of the issues.

The provision of opportunities for such skill development and values exploration implies a broadening of traditional field placements, as well as greater commitment on the part of the profession to student involvement in policy/practice arenas. Increased development could occur in both partisan and non-partisan political activities ranging, for example, from coalition building with the Child Welfare League, to working with a staff person of an elected official. California State University at Sacramento's efforts such as internships with Assemblyperson Polanco are excellent examples of building inroads to politics for social workers.

Greater institutionalizing of political experiences for students should be considered. Local work on political campaigns, via PACE, or participation in Spring "Legislative Days" in Sacramento might serve as field placement projects or class assignments. These kinds of opportunities should not be viewed as voluntary, tangential activities of a few "politically inclined" social workers, but rather as a necessary piece of curriculum, if we, as a profession, have a mission of social change.

In conclusion, there is a need to look at politics and social work within the framework of macro-practice as conceived by the profession and as taught in today's schools of social work. The year 1990 saw a 90% national success rate of PACE endorsements of candidates for public office (Moss, 1991). But we cannot, as a profession, rest on these laurels. Whether the 1990s will bring a "kinder, gentler nation" is still to be seen. And social workers will not be the powerful change agents we can be until "politics" is as endemic to the macro-practitioner's vocabulary as "countertransference" is to the clinician's.

END NOTE

1. Since 1984, Human SERVE has focussed on persuading governors and legislatures to make voter registration automatic when people renew or apply for drivers' licenses, or for welfare or unemployment benefits. This effort has been extremely successful: half of the states now have "motor voter" programs, although states have been less willing to establish voter registration in welfare and unemployment agencies. Legislation is now pending in Congress as of Spring

1992 — the National Voter Registration Act — that would require all states to make voter registration automatic in DMVs, welfare, unemployment, and vocational rehabilitation agencies.

REFERENCES

Abbott, A. *Professional choices: Values at work.* Silver Spring, MD: NASW, 1988.

Almond, G., & Verba, S. *The civic culture.* Princeton, NJ: Princeton University Press, 1963.

Brager, G. Advocacy and political behavior. *Social Work*, 1968, *13*(4), 5-15.

Campbell, A. et al. *The American voter.* New York: Wiley Publications, 1960.

Chambers, C. *Seedtime of reform: American social service and social action, 1918-1933.* Minneapolis: University of Minnesota Press, 1963.

Day, P. *A new history of social welfare.* Englewood Cliffs, NJ: Prentice-Hall, Inc., 1989.

Epstein, I. *Professionalism and social work activism.* Unpublished doctoral dissertation, Columbia University, 1969.

Haynes, K., & Mickelson, J. Politics and social policy: The hidden power base. Paper presented at the Council on Social Work Education, Annual Program Meeting, March, 1985.

Haynes, K. & Mickelson, J. *Affecting change: Social workers in the political arena*, 2nd Ed. New York: Longman, 1991.

Howard, D. Social work and social reform. In C. Kasius (Ed.), *New Directions in Social Work.* New York: Harper, 1954.

Humphreys, N. Teaching politics to today's social work students. Paper presented at the Council on Social Work Education, Annual Program Meeting, Atlanta, March, 1988.

Lane, R. *Political life: Why people get involved in politics.* Glencoe, IL: The Free Press, 1959.

Leiby, J. *A history of social welfare and social work in the United States.* New York: Columbia University Press, 1978.

Leighninger, L. *Social work search for identity.* New York: Greenwood Press, 1987.

Mahaffey, M. Political action in social work. *Encyclopedia of Social Work*, 18th Ed., Vol. 2. Silver Spring, MD: NASW, 1987.

Milbrath, L. *Political participation: How and why do people get involved in politics?* Chicago: Rand McNally, 1965.

Moss, M.S. PACE's election score: 90% victory. *NASW News*, January, 1991.

Piven, F., & Cloward, R. *Why Americans don't vote.* New York: Pantheon Books, 1988.

Reeser, L. *Professional and social activism.* Unpublished doctoral dissertation, Bryn Mawr College, 1986.

Reeser, L. & Epstein, I. Social work attitudes toward poverty and social action: 1968-1984. *Social Service Review*, 1987, *61*, 610-622.

Ribicoff, A. Politics and social workers. *Social Work*, 1962, *7*(4), 3-6.

Schneiderman, L. The political function of social work practice. *Public Welfare*, April, 1970, 198-202.

Thurz, D. Social action as a professional responsibility. *Social Work*, 1966, *2*(3), 12-21.

Verba, S., Nie, N. & Kim, J. *Participation and political equality: A seven nation comparison*. Cambridge, England: Cambridge University Press, 1978.

Wolk, J. Are social workers politically active? *Social Work*, 1981, *26*(4), 285-288.

Woodward, J. & Roper, E. Political activity of American citizens. *American Political Science Review*, 1950, *44*, 872-885.

Infusing a Feminist Analysis into Education for Policy, Planning, and Administration

Judith H. Halseth, EdD

"Women are calling for institutions to recognize their worth fully and to stop assuming that knowledge about men and men's lives necessarily speaks to women and their lives" (American Council on Education, cited in *The Chronicle of Higher Education*, p. A15, 1988).

Creative solutions are needed to address social problems faced by female clients — especially poverty, lack of health care, and underemployment (Hagen & Davis, 1990). Applying a feminist analysis to social welfare policy, program development, and service delivery will continue the process of bringing women, as clients and workers, into the mainstream of a social service system in which decisions are often made in a patriarchal fashion. In a system where a majority of the clients are women and a majority of the workers are women (Abramovitz, 1985), a feminist vision provides a new sensitivity to social problems, policy issues, and organizational processes.

In response to the Council on Social Work Education's mandate systematically to include content on women, schools of social work are increasingly moving toward compliance. Recently, women's voices have stressed the importance of not only adding content on

Dr. Halseth is Associate Professor, School of Social Work, Western Michigan University, Kalamazoo, MI 49008.

An earlier version of this paper was presented at the Annual Program Meeting, Council on Social Work Education, Reno, 1990.

women's issues, but also infusing a feminist analysis into the foundation curriculum for practice, human behavior in the social environment, policy, research, and field education (Bombyk & Graber, 1989; Bricker-Jenkins & Hooyman, 1986; Cummerton, 1986; Davis, 1986; Deanow & Bricker-Jenkins, 1989; Gottlieb & Bombyk, 1987; Kravetz, 1986; Levande, 1989; VanDenBergh & Cooper, 1986). Infusing a feminist analysis into macro-level courses increases awareness of options for gender-sensitive public policies, social programs, and practice models (Bombyk & Chernesky, 1985; Chernesky, 1987; Ewalt, 1987; Weil, 1986), and is the topic of this article.

FEMINIST ANALYSIS

A feminist analysis questions and challenges (a) the distribution of power in society, (b) the dynamic interplay between external systems and internalized beliefs, (c) the social, economic, and political oppression of women, (d) unintended consequences of social welfare policies on women (Deanow & Bricker-Jenkins, 1989), and (e) ways in which societal discrimination affects social service delivery (Gottlieb, 1987).

Evidence of inequalities related to the power differential between women and men and the societal discrimination against women has been documented elsewhere (Kanter, 1977; Miller, J. B., 1986). This inequality is currently seen in increasing levels of poverty among women and children — particularly among women who are not in a relationship where they are economically dependent on a man — among women of color (Lefkowitz & Withorn, 1986; Sidel, 1986), and among older women (O'Grady-LeShane, 1990). "Punishing these women for their manlessness is a major patriarchal function of the social welfare system" (Miller, D. C., 1990, p. 23).

A feminist lens helps illuminate aspects of public policy and social programs affecting women which may be misunderstood, underestimated, or denied (Abramovitz, 1988; Segal, 1989; Spakes, 1989). And a feminist lens may encourage decision-makers toward developing new and creative views and frameworks for alleviating problems such as the increasing level of poverty among women and children.

THE STATUS OF GENDER BALANCING

Social work educators appear to be adding content on women and on minorities, in response to CSWE mandates, and perhaps in some cases as the result of a raised consciousness on perspectives previously ignored or forgotten. However, resources and content added to a course outline or syllabus may consist of only one article known to the professor — a token — added in compliance, or perhaps out of guilt. The token article may, unwittingly, contribute to further perpetuation of stereotypes, or ignore recent research and literature on, for example, the new psychology of women, or the impact of public policy on women. Or, the professor may invite a guest speaker to cover the topic of "women" for the semester, and allow the remainder of the semester's work to remain relatively unaffected by a concern for issues raised by a pro-feminist consciousness (Levande & Halseth, 1986).

Almost a decade ago, Kravetz (1982) predicted, "to a large degree, faculty readiness and ability to challenge and modify their own sexist values will determine the extent to which content on women will be fully integrated into social work courses" (p. 47).

Work by faculty at Hunter College and other schools of social work has documented the need and has encouraged efforts to "incorporate gender variables and new grounded knowledge about women" (Burden & Gottlieb, 1987, p. 7). The Hunter College project (Abramovitz & Helly, 1987) on gender balancing noted that traditional assumptions about women continue to drive the knowledge-base of theory and research and may lead to gender bias in service delivery. The Hunter project concluded that while some educators may be aware of new scholarship on women, they "have lacked the time and academic incentives to study it, to identify key issues, and to incorporate the material into their courses" (Abramovitz & Helly, 1987, pp. 3-4).

Faculty development is an important step in shifting from "the way we've always taught it" into a new framework for viewing and reviewing the macro-curriculum. The process of developing a pro-feminist consciousness and infusing a feminist analysis involves moving beyond looking at a list of suggested themes and resources and into reading, thinking, listening, and discussing these ideas.

The next step involves rethinking and revising course objectives, student assignments, and the task and process of class sessions in all macro-areas. The following section addresses these issues.

A GENDER-SENSITIVE MACRO CURRICULUM

The curriculum for policy, planning, and administration generally includes courses which prepare students for roles in the planning, design, and management of social welfare policies, organizations, and services.

The second part of this article identifies and addresses seven components of the macro-curriculum: policy, planning and program development, community organizing and development, research and program evaluation, administration/management, field education, and the learning environment. To assist in reviewing and revising the curriculum with a gender lens, suggestions are offered for readings, activities, and course assignments. The seven components of the curriculum, as well as the readings and assignments, tend to overlap and affect each other in a complementary and synergistic fashion.

Policy

At the heart of the policy sequence is the examination and analysis of policies and programs at agency, community, state, and federal levels which may inhibit or promote self-sufficiency in female clients. "Public policies and practice models must reflect the differing needs of women and men for services" (Hagen & Davis, 1990, p. 16). Sensitizing students and agency people to question and challenge policy issues and their impact on women may empower social workers to take a more proactive role in policy development.

Areas of concern include poverty, access to health care, homelessness, mental illness, violence against females, chemical dependency, employment opportunities and expectations, reproductive rights, and responsibility for care of children and elders.

For the topic of women and welfare, the following resources incorporate a gender lens to analyze the effects of social policies, social programs, and social work practice models on women.

Miller (1989, 1990) analyzes new welfare-to-work programs and concludes that they indicate little success in getting women off welfare or out of poverty. She discusses how the failure of these programs is functional to patriarchy, capitalism, and white supremacy. Abramovitz (1986, 1988) analyzes how the family ethic and "profamily" platforms have perpetuated punitive welfare approaches toward women and have exacerbated female poverty. Hagen and Davis (1990) use a conceptual framework built on role equity and role change. They offer principles of social action and social work practice in conservative times. Others who have examined these welfare policy issues from a feminist perspective include Burden (1987), Gordon (1990), Lefkowitz & Withorn (1986), Nichols-Casebolt & Klawitter (1990), Segal (1989), Sidel (1986), and Spakes (1989).

In addition to these suggestions, *Affilia: Journal of Women and Social Work* provides a rich resource of feminist scholarship and contains many articles appropriate for macro-courses.

The following options for assignments can specifically ask students to apply a gender lens.

1. Analyze a legislative proposal affecting women, "e.g., a state or local bill, government ordinance, or a policy established by a local controlling board of concern to the student's agency" (Flynn, 1989b, p. 2).
2. Propose and develop a policy—at the agency, community, state, or federal level—to address a problem or situation affecting women.
3. Write a paper or present a panel discussion in class, perhaps composed of students, consumers of services, and agency representatives, "identifying the extent to which racism, sexism and classism are evident in social welfare policies and programs" (Flynn, 1989a p. 2).
4. Design and lead an exercise in dyads or small groups, related to assumptions, issues, or public policies affecting women. This consciousness-raising activity could include open-ended statements such as (a) I think the hardest thing about being a homeless woman would be . . . , (b) An experience I had with limited resources . . . , (c) I think a woman on welfare . . . ,

(d) I wish the welfare system . . . , and (e) My idea for improving access to health care for women is. . . . Then, process the activity with a general group discussion.

In addition, students can be encouraged to understand that women need to be more actively involved in public policy decision making so that policies benefitting women will be enacted and implemented. Equity in decision making around gender issues in public policy can occur only when women adequately represent their proportion of the population (Sarri et al., 1987).

Planning and Program Development

These topics focus on improved program development and delivery of services to female clients which empower them to overcome societal oppression and dependence upon public assistance.

For problems such as homelessness and chemical dependency, programs for women are too often built on models designed for men. Benda and Dattalo (1990) examined the relationship between homelessness and gender, and found that while men may become homeless after years of crime and alcohol abuse, homeless women are more likely to have abused nonprescription drugs. Benda and Dattalo then developed recommendations for programs addressing, from a feminist perspective, the unique needs of women.

In an analysis of four battered women's programs in Appalachia, Tice (1990) cites the programs' "commitment to the models of feminist social work practice of empowerment and advocacy" and their challenge to "the *status quo* of male privilege" (p. 98).

In an assignment to design a program, service delivery system, needs evaluation, or program evaluation, the planner can explicitly "identify the variations in conceptions and meanings of need among women, minorities, and ethnic groups" (Pawlak, 1989, p. 1). The setting could be either the student's field placement or another community program. The following questions could help guide the student's design: (a) what aspects of the program may enhance or diminish the program's effectiveness in meeting the needs of the female clients? (b) does the program, service delivery system, or treatment in some way "blame the victim"? (c) how could the program be reconceptualized to avoid blaming the client for failing to overcome the constraints in her social situation that block personal and social effectiveness? (d) how can the program empower women clients? and (e) what mobilizing of resources and advocacy for clients (Dodd & Gutierrez, 1990) are important for successful outcomes for clients?

Community Organizing and Developing

> The feminist vision in community practice is one of social, personal, and political transformation. . . . As feminism unites the political and the personal, community practice is the means of moving social work from case to cause and from private troubles to public concerns. (Weil, 1986, p. 207)

Amidei (1989) and Martin and Chernesky (1989) recently observed that social workers are more likely to mobilize around their own professional self-interests on an issue such as licensure, than to organize and lobby on behalf of legislation and public policies which directly affect the welfare of clients.

Chandler (1986) points out that one component of social work education and social work practice focuses on an individual's intrapsychic or interpersonal problems, with the worker assisting the client in coping or changing. She continues:

> Another component attempts to examine the systems that negatively impinge on individuals and intervene by altering, changing, or restructuring those systems, institutions, and environments that may directly or indirectly prevent individual, group, or community self-actualization. . . . Feminists see the necessity for bringing about both types of change to achieve equality for women and all oppressed people. (pp. 158, 161)

Additional resources on community organizing, developing, and empowerment are found in (a) the bibliography from The Women Organizers' Collective at Hunter College (Joseph, Lob, McLaughlin Mizrahi, Peterson, Rosenthal, & Sugarman, 1989) which identifies references with a feminist perspective, and (b) papers from the 1988 Symposium of the Association on Community Organization and Social Administration (ACOSA) (Weil & Kruzich, 1990).

Students studying community organization can move beyond looking at an individual woman needing help in solving her problems, toward proposing and facilitating change at a wider level. Assignments can focus on examining social justice issues in the community which affect women and on designing strategies for change.

Weil (1986) suggests course content and assignments for community and macro-practice courses. Faculty and students can examine alternative services for women, promote advocacy activities, and develop positive links between alternative services and mainstream services. Weil suggests students need exposure to feminist approaches and to experiential learning strategies which include value clarification, leadership styles, and role conflict. She also recommends that students become involved in planning, organizing, and action tasks—preferably out in the community where they can participate and gain experience in community practice (Weil, 1986).

Research and Program Evaluation

Research and research findings permeate the entire social work curriculum. Sensitivity to gender bias in research and support of gender-sensitive research which informs social policies and programs offer challenges for the 1990s. Students, faculty, and agency personnel can become more aware of the problem noted by Abramovitz (1985), that "social welfare literature has focused on male recipients while generalizing its findings to women" (p. 15), which may result in distorting or ignoring the actual experiences of females.

Qualitative research methods form an important component of gender-sensitive research courses. To move away from the guise of objectivity, and into a partnership of discovery, Cummerton (1986) suggests the following:

> Feminine research has been conceptualized as being process oriented, allowing participants to define themselves and their experiences, focusing on the growth of researchers and participants, and leading to action and social change (p. 97).

Davis (1989) emphasizes the importance of "research with women, discovering the reality of women, and not the reality of the researchers" (p. 558).

In research courses and in courses that use research findings, students and faculty can look for evidence of inclusion of women in the study, if the findings are applied to women. Students can look for possible stereotypical assumptions about the roles or attributes of women and men. And they can consider how those assumptions affect the research design as well as interpretation of findings. In the design of social services and social welfare policies, such assumptions and research findings may perpetuate oppression or powerlessness of women.

Students, faculty, and agency personnel can be encouraged to design and conduct research on women, using qualitative methods or combining qualitative and quantitative methods, which encourage participants to describe their needs, experiences, and ideas for problem solving. This can effectively blur the boundaries between the "expert" and the "subject," and may lead to action, social change, and policies and programs which empower women.

Administration/Management

One purpose of a gender-sensitive macro track is to support strategies for fostering the participation of women in leadership roles in social work.

"Feminist social workers justifiably have criticized the ways in which macro-practice has neglected the contributions of women" (Hyde, 1989, p. 145). Faculty, field instructors, and students can become more sensitive to the significance of gender differences and sex-role socialization in the group and organizational behavior of women and men around such issues as achievement, affiliation, use of power, and gender composition (Kravetz, 1982; Savage, 1987).

Studies on gender differences in leadership styles suggest that the management style of women is different from the management style of men (Helgesen, 1990; Hooyman & Cunningham, 1986; Loden, 1985). "Women bring to their administrative positions a unique view and understanding of women's experience of caring and, in so doing, may be more effective managers" (Chernesky & Bombyk,

1988, p. 48). Martin and Chernesky (1989) advocate moving "society away from masculinist values that emphasize hierarchy over egalitarianism, competition over cooperation, rugged individualism over nurturance, and conflict over peace" (pp. 134-135).

Stokes (1986) warns against using a "deficiency model" in training and development programs for women. She points out that using masculine behavior as the model for standards of professional behavior has resulted in viewing women as inherently deficient.

> The unfortunate consequence is that attention is paid more often to repairing the presumed deficiencies than to constructing a favorable work climate in which the individual talents and skills of women can be recognized, displayed, and used (p. 18).

The American Council on Education (ACE) (cited in *The Chronicle of Higher Education*, 1988) acknowledges the importance and strengths of women as leaders.

> They [women] are calling for institutions to start systematically educating women for leadership in society. And they are calling for institutions to stop expecting them to give up their own strengths as women to become part of the male system. (p. A15)

In her curriculum model for women in administration, Weil (1987) advises that women need to emerge with the following:

1. Competencies in the process and task skills needed for managing people and information.
2. Knowledge of and abilities to handle sexism and discrimination in the workplace.
3. Knowledge of various models of organizational structures and cultures.
4. Knowledge of how to develop a managerial style appropriate to the organizational setting and culture.
5. Knowledge of and skills in organizational change processes in order to build programs and organizations more supportive of women as clients, workers, and administrators. (pp. 106-107)

The curriculum can also deal with "the dual impacts of racism and sexism . . . and career planning/career management" (Healy, Havens, & Chin, 1990, p. 92).

The following assignment could sensitize students to issues for women in leadership roles: (a) look at the problems of sexism in leadership in a human service organization; (b) what are the unique experiences of and unique demands on women in management? (c) what could improve the climate for women? and (d) using literature and your own ideas, develop strategies for use at the individual, interpersonal, and organizational/structural levels.

Through curriculum development and through encouragement of area human service organizations, schools of social work can strive to improve the climate for women who aspire to or who are already in leadership positions (Halseth, 1988).

Field Education

Field education manuals, objectives, assignments, and evaluation instruments can explicitly include items sensitive to gender issues (Garner, Graber, & Gottlieb, 1989). Faculty can initiate changes leading to "nonsexist field-based learning conditions" (Berkun, 1984). The following goals are suggested for macro field placements:

1. Enable students to understand the impact of societal values and social-demographic changes on women's roles, responsibilities, and needs for service.
2. Enable students to formulate a comprehensive assessment of the appropriateness of existing services for women. (Davidson, Martin, & Haffey, 1988, p. 2)

Dodd and Gutierrez (1990) offer a framework which the student could incorporate in an assessment of appropriateness of existing services for women. Using a "power perspective on community practice" (p. 73), and in the context of providing gender-sensitive services, they offer five specific techniques for empowering clients. Within a collaborative helping relationship, preferably using small group work, they suggest (a) accepting the client's definition of the problem, (b) identifying and building upon existing strengths,

(c) raising the client's awareness of issues of power imbalance, (d) teaching specific skills, and (e) mobilizing resources or advocating for clients (pp. 71-73).

The macro student can assess and plan how these techniques could more effectively be incorporated into the services offered by the agency.

Suggested evaluation items for macro students in a field placement include the following:

1. Assists in the development of resources to meet the needs of women and minorities.
2. Uses communication which is devoid of sexist language.
3. Demonstrates knowledge and understanding of research and practice principles regarding women. (Garner, Graber & Gottlieb, 1989, pp. 4-5)

The field education director, faculty liaisons, and a field education advisory committee can develop goals and sample evaluation items which encourage macro students, field instructors, and faculty liaisons to view practice methods, client services, and administrative policies and practices through a gender lens. This can provide an essential link between classroom and agency in promoting gender-sensitive practice.

The Learning Environment

As an integral part of a gender-sensitive macro curriculum, the learning environment — in the offices and halls, the classroom, and the field agencies — should be sensitive to the issues addressed above. "Egalitarian relationships need to be modeled among faculty and between faculty and students" (Kissman & Davis-Sacks, 1990, p. 8). The faculty as a whole can address the importance of adequate numbers of women faculty and women field instructors to serve as role models. Faculty can also discuss ways to promote a gender-sensitive climate in the school.

The "chilly classroom climate" (Hall & Sandler, 1982) refers to ways in which women's experiences in the classroom may reflect subtle or not-so-subtle sex discrimination. Attending to both task and process in the classroom, and valuing diversity in style and ways of learning, may enhance the learning experience for all students.

Feminist social workers point out that the means are as important as the end. Freeman (1986) suggests that the classroom climate can value process equally with product. "How one pursues a goal is as important as the accomplishment of the goal" (VanDenBergh & Cooper, 1986, p. 6).

In addition to stretching outside traditional ways of viewing the impact of social policy and social programs on females, the students and faculty can also stretch outside traditional ways of meeting course requirements. To support this, faculty and agency people can build in opportunities for "negotiated assignments, team-based assignments" (Kissman & Davis-Sacks, 1990, pp. 10-11), experiential learning, group process, collective decision making, feedback, and empowerment of women.

CONCLUSION

Effective social work practice, at micro and macro levels, "requires the empowerment of clients to lead independent, productive, and emotionally satisfying lives" (Burden & Gottlieb, 1987, p. 6). Infusing a feminist analysis into the curriculum for policy, planning, and administration encourages social work educators, students, and agency practitioners to attend to gender variables, incorporate new grounded knowledge about women, and influence policy development, program design, and service delivery more supportive of women as clients, workers, and administrators.

REFERENCES

Abramovitz, M. The family ethic and the female pauper: A new perspective on public aid and Social Security programs. *Journal of Social Work Education*, 1985, *21*(2), 15-26.

Abramovitz, M. *Regulating the lives of women: Social welfare policy from colonial times to the present*. Boston: South End Press, 1988.

Abramovitz, M. Social policy and the female pauper: The family ethic and the U. S. welfare state. In N. VanDenBergh & L.B. Cooper (Eds.), *Feminist visions for social work*. Silver Spring, MD: NASW, 1986.

Abramovitz, M. & Helly, D.O. (Eds.). *Report on a project to integrate scholar-*

ship on women in the professional curriculum at Hunter College. New York: Hunter College, 1987.

American Council on Education. *The new agenda of women for higher education*. Quoted in *The Chronicle of Higher Education*, January 27, 1988, A15.

Amidei, N. *When budgets drive policy*. Speech presented at the NASW Conference, San Francisco, 1989.

Benda, B.B. & Dattalo, P. Homeless women and men: Their problems and use of services. *Affilia: Journal of Women and Social Work*, 1990, *5*(3), 50-82.

Berkun, C.S. Women and the field experience: Toward a model of nonsexist field-based learning conditions. *Journal of Education for Social Work*, 1984, *20*(3), 5-12.

Bombyk, M.J. & Chernesky, R.H. Conventional cutback leadership and the quality of the workplace: Is Beta better? *Administration in Social Work*, 1985, *9*(3), 47-56.

Bombyk, M. & Graber, H. *The "F. . . ." word in social work: Is feminism a dirty word?* Discussion led at the APM of the Council on Social Work Education, Chicago, 1989.

Bricker-Jenkins, M. & Hooyman, N. (Eds.). *Not for women only: Social work practice for a feminist future*. Silver Spring, MD: NASW, 1986.

Burden, D. Women and social policy. In D. Burden & N. Gottlieb (Eds.), *The woman client: Providing human services in a changing world*. New York: Tavistock Publications, 1987.

Burden, D. & Gottlieb, N. (Eds.). *The woman client: Providing human services in a changing world*. New York: Tavistock Publications, 1987.

Chandler, S.M. The hidden feminist agenda in social development. In N. VanDenBergh & L.B. Cooper (Eds.), *Feminist visions for social work*. Silver Spring, MD: NASW, 1986.

Chernesky, R.H. Women and management: From optimism to pessimism. *Affilia*, 1987, *2*(2), 69-71.

Chernesky, R.H. & Bombyk, M.J. Women's ways and effective management. *Affilia*, 1988, *3*(1), 48-61.

Cummerton, J.M. A feminist perspective on research: What does it help us see? In N. VanDenBergh & L.B. Cooper (Eds.), *Feminist visions for social work*. Silver Spring, MD: NASW, 1986.

Davidson, K., Martin, M. & Haffey, M. *A guide for applying a gender lens to field instruction for clinical practice*. Paper presented at the APM of the Council on Social Work Education, Atlanta, 1988.

Davis, L.V. Empirical clinical practice from a feminist perspective: A response to Ivanoff, Robinson, and Blythe. *Social Work*, 1989, *34*, 557-558.

Davis, L.V. A feminist approach to social work research. *Affilia*, 1986, *1*(1), 32-47.

Deanow, C.G. & Bricker-Jenkins, M. *Infusing women's content and a feminist analysis into foundation curriculum*. Paper presented at the APM of the Council on Social Work Education, Chicago, 1989.

Dodd, P. & Gutierrez, L. Preparing students for the future: A power perspective on community practice. *Administration in Social Work*, 1990, *14*(2), 63-78.

Ewalt, P.L. *Women in social work administration*. Paper presented at the APM of the Council on Social Work Education, St. Louis, 1987.

Flynn, J.P. Foundations of social welfare policy: Course outline. Kalamazoo: Western Michigan University, 1989a.

Flynn, J.P. Seminar in social welfare policy practice: Course outline. Kalamazoo: Western Michigan University, 1989b.

Freeman, M.L. *The influences of feminist identification on views of women's issues*. Paper presented at the APM of the Council on Social Work Education, Miami, 1986.

Garner, D., Graber, H. & Gottlieb, N. *Guidelines for incorporating gender issues in field practice manuals*. Paper presented at the NASW Conference, San Francisco, 1989.

Gordon, L. (Ed.). *Women, the state, and welfare*. Madison: University of Wisconsin Press, 1990.

Gottlieb, N. *Service correctives for gender bias*. Paper presented at the APM of the Council on Social Work Education, St. Louis, 1987.

Gottlieb, N. & Bombyk, M. Strategies for strengthening feminist research. *Affilia*, 1987, *2*(2), 23-35.

Hagen, J.L. & Davis, L.V. *Working with women: Social policy and social work practice issues for the 1990s*. Paper presented at the APM of the Council on Social Work Education, Reno, 1990.

Hall, R. & Sandler, B. *The classroom climate: A chilly one for women?* Washington, DC: Association of American Colleges, 1982.

Halseth, J.H. *Designing a leadership institute for women: Initial steps*. Paper presented at the APM of the Council on Social Work Education, Atlanta, 1988.

Healy, L.M., Havens, C.M. & Chin, A. Preparing women for human service administration: Building on experience. *Administration in Social Work*, 1990, *14*(2), 79-94.

Helgesen, S. *The female advantage: Women's ways of leadership*. New York: Doubleday, 1990.

Hooyman, N.R. & Cunningham, R. An alternative administrative style. In N. VanDenBergh & L.B. Cooper (Eds.), *Feminist visions for social work*. Silver Spring, MD: NASW, 1986.

Hyde, C. A feminist model for macro-practice: Promises and problems. *Administration in Social Work*, 1989, *13*(3/4), 145-181.

Joseph, B., Lob, S., McLaughlin, P., Mizrahi, T., Peterson, J., Rosenthal, B. & Sugarman, F. *Women organizers: A beginning collection of references and resources*. New York: ECCO/WOC, Hunter College School of Social Work, 1989.

Kanter, R.M. *Men and women of the corporation*. New York: Basic Books, 1977.

Kissman, K. & Davis-Sacks, M.L. *Implementing feminist-based service technol-*

ogies: Implications for social work education. Paper presented at the APM of the Council on Social Work Education, Reno, 1990.

Kravetz, D. An overview of content on women for the social work curriculum. *Journal of Education for Social Work*, 1982, *18*(2), 42-49.

Kravetz, D. Women and mental health. In N. VanDenBergh & L.B. Cooper (Eds.), *Feminist visions for social work.* Silver Spring, MD: NASW, 1986.

Lefkowitz, R. & Withorn, A. (Eds.). *For crying out loud: Women and poverty in the United States.* New York: Pilgrim Press, 1986.

Levande, D.I. *The developmental needs of older women: Exploring the theoretical chasm.* Paper presented at the APM of the Council on Social Work Education, Chicago, 1989.

Levande, D.I. & Halseth, J.H. *From "add women and stir" to curriculum transformation.* Paper presented at the APM of the Council on Social Work Education, Miami, 1986.

Loden, M. *Feminine leadership or how to succeed in business without being one of the boys.* New York: Times Books, 1985.

Martin, P.Y. & Chernesky, R.H. Women's prospects for leadership in social welfare: A political economy perspective. *Administration in Social Work*, 1989, *13*(3/4), 117-143.

Miller, D.C. Poor women and work programs: Back to the future. *Affilia*, 1989, *4*(1), 9-21.

Miller, D.C. *Women and social welfare: A feminist analysis.* New York: Praeger, 1990.

Miller, J.B. *Toward a new psychology of women* (2nd ed.). Boston: Beacon, 1986.

Nichols-Casebolt, A. & Klawitter, M. Child support enforcement reform: Can it reduce the welfare dependency of families of never-married mothers? *Journal of Sociology & Social Welfare*, 1990, *17*(3), 23-54.

O'Grady-LeShane, R. Older women and poverty. *Social Work*, 1990, *35*, 422-424.

Pawlak, E.J. Program planning: Course outline. Kalamazoo: Western Michigan University, 1989.

Sarri, R., et al. *Women in Michigan: A statistical portrait.* Lansing: Michigan Women's Commission, 1987.

Savage, A. Integrating additional gender sensitive material into an administration course for non-administration majors in a social work program. In M. Abramovitz & D.O. Helly (Eds.), *Report on a project to integrate scholarship on women into the professional curriculum at Hunter College.* New York: Hunter College, 1987.

Segal, E.A. Welfare reform: Help for poor women and children? *Affilia*, 1989, *4*(3), 42-50.

Sidel, R. *Women and children last: The plight of poor women in affluent America.* New York: Penguin Books, 1986.

Spakes, P. Reshaping the goals of family policy: Sexual equality, not protection. *Affilia*, 1989, *4*(3), 7-24.

Stokes, J. Deficiencies among women: A compelling but faulty premise for professional development. *Journal of NAWDAC*, 1986, *49*(3), 14-19.

Tice, K.W. A case study of battered women's shelters in Appalachia. *Affilia*, 1990, *5*(3), 83-100.

VanDenBergh, N. & Cooper, L.B. Introduction. In N. VanDenBergh & L B. Cooper (Eds.), *Feminist visions for social work*. Silver Spring, MD: NASW, 1986.

Weil, M. Women, community, and organizing. In N. VanDenBergh & L.B. Cooper (Eds.), *Feminist visions for social work*. Silver Spring, MD: NASW, 1986.

Weil, M. Women in administration: Curriculum and strategies. In D. Burden & N. Gottlieb (Eds.), *The woman client: Providing human services in a changing world*. New York: Tavistock Publications, 1987.

Weil, M. & Kruzich, J. (Eds.). Empowerment issues in administrative and community practice. *Administration in Social Work*, 1990, *14*(2), 1-12.

Index

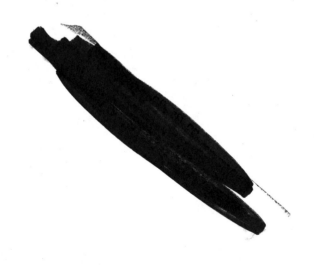